Enjoy the
book!
Carolene

While the depth of her knowledge is tremendously impressive, what changed my life was her ability to explain in a straightforward manner, a subject that I previously found intimidating. When people hear the word vegan, they usually think of a sparse diet that will deprive them of everything delicious, but this wonderful book is full of enticing recipes that soon make you lose you cravings for unhealthy alternatives. I urge anyone interested in living a healthier lifestyle to read this book.

—Marcie Weithorn, Miami, Florida

Caroline's influence in my life was the greatest when I needed someone to educate me about how what I was eating had affected my health, and I found myself prepared to make the change to a more plant based diet. The effects were immediate. I had more energy and vitality and felt in control and life changed for the better.

Helping others live their best lives through healthy choices is what comes naturally to Caroline. It is her passion that is forever inspiring to anyone who has the privilege of meeting her.

—Anna Barten, Sydney, Australia

I have known Caroline for over twenty years, and her knowledge and expertise in the health and nutrition field has been an inspiration to not only me and my family, but everyone who knows her. This book is extremely informative and I find the content very inspiring. I look forward to sampling the recipes, and increasing my intake of plant based foods.

—Andy Stuart, President & CEO Norwegian Cruise Line

I have been an endurance based athlete most of my life, and as such have subscribed to the notion that nutrition is vital to success. From college hockey to running marathons and competing in triathlons to summiting some of the highest peaks of the world, proper nutrition is key. After reading numerous books since 1985, I have finally found one that encompasses lifestyle recipes for both performance and health. I will be utilizing the recipes found in the pages of Caroline's book as I prepare to climb Everest and K2.

—Godspeed, David Kestner, Anchorage, Alaska

With 20 years of expertise in health and nutrition, Caroline Hale, has long known the benefits of a plant-based diet. This book is filled with delicious, easy to follow recipes and will provide a wonderful pathway to optimal health.

—Emmanuela Wolloch MD, holistic gynecologist

When I decided to go Plant Strong, I was fortunate enough to find Caroline, and she made my transition a pleasure and full of discovery. Her creations are delicious and so nutritional.

—Jason Callender, Albany, Nassau

I work in the field of health and fitness, so I understand how important it is to fuel the body with the right nutrients. Caroline is a wealth of knowledge when it comes to health and nutrition. I consider myself fortunate to have her close-by to consult with for me and my clients. This book is amazing!

—Verena Koefler, Personal Trainer, Miami Beach, Florida

Caroline has guided me with my nutritional needs for nearly eight years. She has helped me to look and feel the best I can at my age, and I am very grateful for being fortunate enough to have her in my life. I am very excited to see her help and guide others as she has guided me.

—Natasha Dubarry, Miami Beach, Florida

I was very fortunate to find Caroline Hale, who's nutritional advice was extremely effective in addressing my concerns.

With Caroline's guidance, I began a strictly whole food, plant based diet by following Caroline's Live Simply Plant Based lifestyle, and within 4 months I lost 22 pounds, my blood pressure was perfect, my cholesterol level was in the 150 range, my LDL and triglycerides were normal, my HDL increased and my liver enzymes returned to a normal level. Additionally, my blood sugar and hA1c returned to normal along with my PSA level.

People ask me if I'm tired, lethargic or have no energy since I'm not eating animal protein. Actually, I feel much healthier, and more energetic.

I am so happy with my results, I simply want to share my experience in the hopes that it will help others.

—Scott Stupay, Washington DC

Caroline was a life saver in helping me, so I have extreme confidence in her abilities where health and nutrition are concerned. Congratulations on the book and I look forward to trying these new and enticing recipes.

—Cathy Imburgia, Miami, Florida

Caroline has always been ahead of the nutrition curve. Her passion and enthusiasm coupled with her extensive training and knowledge will always shine through to teach and motivate people to obtain a healthier lifestyle. This book is an extension of what she lives, and I cannot wait to incorporate some of these delicious recipes into my lifestyle.

—Shelley Witiak, Orlando, Florida

The Sustainable Lifestyle for Optimal Health

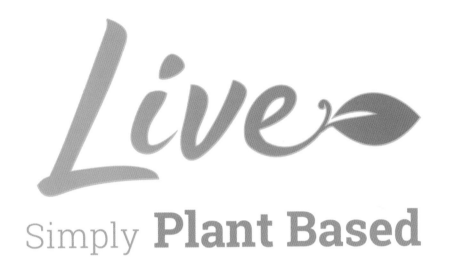

Simply Plant Based

Caroline Hale

VALEWORTH MEDIA, LLC

Published by Valeworth Media, LLC

ISBN: 978-0-9998422-0-1

Photo credits: Food photos on the cover and pages xvi, xx,
xxiv, xxvi, 32, 42, 84, 86, 88, 91, 94, 97, 99, 100, 102, 104, 105,
116, 118, 123, 129, 137, 140, 142, 147, 151, 154, 156, 159,
161, 162, 164, 167, 169, 170, 172, 174, 179, 181, 185, 187, 190,
191, 194, 203, 205, 207, 209, 214, 215, 217, 219, 225, 230,
249, 255, 258, 266, 268, 269, 270, 276 by RM Studio Corp.
Photos on pages 107, 131, 149, 173, 188, 193, 210, 227, 229,
235, 238, 257, 273, by the author. Page 294, Shutterstock ©
marilyn barbone, page 242 Shutterstock © Elena Veselova.

Edited by Mikel Benton
Book Design by DesignForBooks.com

Printed in the U.S.A.

DISCLAIMER

This publication contains the opinions and ideas of the author. It
is sold with the understanding that the author and publisher are
not engaged in rendering health services in the book. You should
consult your own medical and health providers as appropriate
before adopting any of the suggestions in this book or drawing
inferences from it.

The author and publisher specifically disclaim all responsibility
for any liability, loss or risk, personal or otherwise, which is
incurred as a consequence, directly or indirectly, of the use and
application of any of the contents of this book.

Contents

11 Main Dishes   165

12 Dressings, Sauces, and Toppings   231

13 Snacks   255

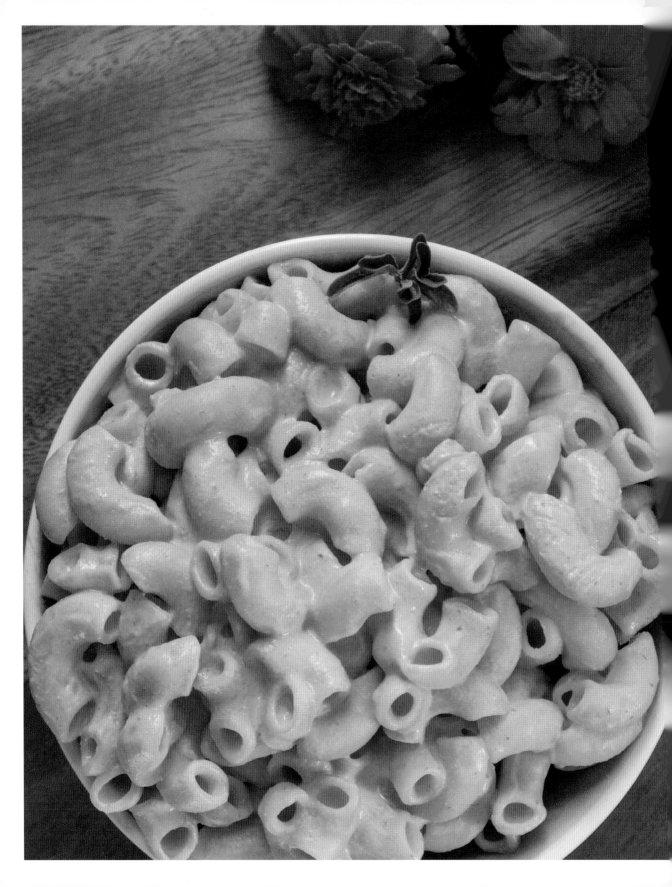

Preface

My passion for discovery led me to write this book. As an accomplished young athlete, I thought I was unstoppable, until I had to deal with health issues that were beyond my age. I began suffering with gynecological problems such as ovarian cysts and endometriosis. In my quest to get to the root of these problems, I discovered a direct correlation to my diet being high in animal protein, and my living environment being chemically toxic. Research led me to discover that a plant-based lifestyle could be the answer to reversing my condition.

At seventeen, I was told by a gynecologist that I had a hormonal imbalance, and was prescribed the contraceptive pill, which the doctor assured me would help my condition. However, the prescription did not help. In fact, my condition worsened as ovarian cysts grew, causing ever-increasing pain. After my first laparoscopy, I was given another prescription at age nineteen. This time the prescription was for a male steroid, which forced my body to shut down its production of estrogen, mimicking menopause.

After being put through many more surgical procedures, and treated with the usual pharmaceutical approaches to illness, I began researching natural alternatives, along with educating myself in health and fitness. I became certified in personal training and yoga. I realized that I would probably achieve better results by treating my body as a whole, rather than treating each individual symptom

I thought I was unstoppable, until I had to deal with health issues that were beyond my age.

in isolation. By adopting a healthy, pharmaceutical-free lifestyle, a healthier plant-based, whole food diet, and a proper exercise regiment, I could "re-set" my body and eliminate the potentially adverse effects of the typical diet and lifestyle I had regressed to. I threw all of the pharmaceutical prescriptions into the garbage and went back to school to educate myself on the benefits of a holistic lifestyle.

I completed a degree in natural health and a doctorate in naturopathy with a concentration in nutrition. Naturopathy, the foundation on which all methods of natural therapies are based, is a system of healing that allows us to follow our natural instincts, enabling the healing power of nature to take place. I believe that the majority of allopathic medicine has strayed so far from nature that it has complicated the body's entire system of healing. The combination of natural therapies, such as nutrition, clean water, fresh air, sunlight, and plants and herbs as medicines, are all included in the field of naturopathy.

I opened my nutritional consulting practice in 2004 and began assisting other people who were not getting the answers they so desperately needed from their physicians. I became certified in plant-based nutrition, expanding my knowledge in the health and nutrition field. I have nearly twenty years of experience in health and nutrition, and thirty years in health and fitness.

I wrote this book because I wanted to reach a population larger than those I am able to help in my local community. I want everyone to be aware of the dangers of a high-animal-protein diet and the benefits of a plant-based lifestyle. Every little change in achieving your plant-based lifestyle is a step toward greater health and vitality. The motivation for me to write this book comes from the desire to share the knowledge and expertise gained through my unique combination of personal health research, extensive education, and practical, hands-on experience from my health, nutrition, and fitness consulting practices.

Every little change in achieving your plant-based lifestyle is a step toward greater health and vitality.

This book aims to provide you with the information and tools to:

- Increase energy
- Increase mental focus
- Increase immunity
- Boost metabolism
- Improve well-being
- Improve sleep
- Reduce stress
- Reduce cravings
- Speed exercise recovery
- Prevent and reverse disease
- Improve overall health

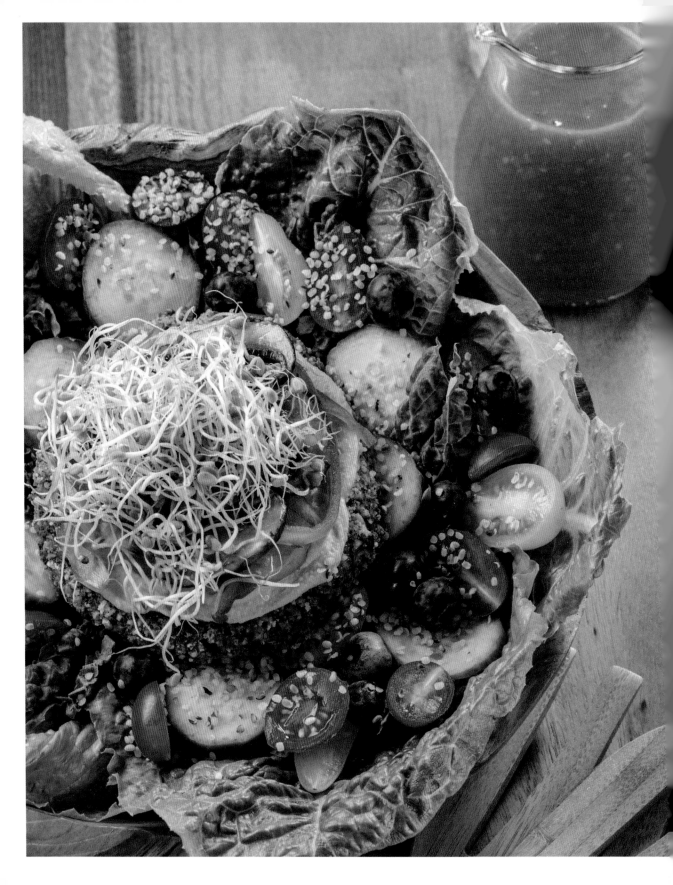

Introduction

ive Simply Plant-Based is an easily readable compendium of the knowledge I have obtained through extensive education, and years of first-hand research and observation of the positive effects on the human body of a whole food, plant-based diet.

This book will inform you of the multitude of benefits that can be experienced by adopting a whole food, plant-based diet. Armed with the knowledge that follows, you may find that you see the common-sense reasons that will encourage you to adapt this lifestyle. *Live Simply Plant-Based* is about understanding the benefits of proper nutrition and the healthy lifestyle you can easily achieve by consistently making informed food choices for the benefit of your health. This lifestyle is sustainable and will help you to achieve optimal health, by substantially increasing energy levels, boosting immunity, and helping to increase mental focus. Cravings will be reduced as you boost metabolism, lose weight naturally, and benefit from increased immunity. Learn to reduce stress, improve sleep, reverse and prevent disease, and potentially lengthen your life.

Chapter one explains the many health benefits of following a whole food, plant-based lifestyle. We will look at the leading causes of death, what increases our risks of these diseases, and what can be done to minimize the risks. I have also included a few success stories of people who have reversed disease by adhering to a whole

Learn to reduce stress, improve sleep, reverse and prevent disease, and potentially lengthen your life.

food, plant-based diet. We will look at stress-reducing practices and learn how to incorporate them into this healthy, sustainable lifestyle.

Chapter two takes a close look at the dangers of consuming high-animal-protein/low-carbohydrate diets. You will find explanations of why these diets are unhealthy, how they affect the body, and why they are not sustainable in the long term. I list healthy plant proteins and amino acids, and explain why plant proteins combined with complex carbohydrates are a much healthier alternative to animal-protein-based diets. We will also take a look at some common illnesses associated with the overconsumption of animal protein, and why humans do not need cow's milk to obtain sufficient calcium.

Chapter three examines the acid/alkaline balance in the human body and why this is important to balancing pH homeostasis. I have created lists of acid-forming and alkaline-forming foods, and I explain the health benefits of consuming a predominantly alkaline diet, including why we should minimize the consumption of acid-forming foods.

Chapter four touches on genetically modified organisms (GMOs), and the potential dangers of consuming these foods. I discuss neurotoxic substances (excitotoxins) in foods and the health-related concerns linked to them. I also touch on a potentially dangerous chemical found in many foods and drinks that are stocked in our grocery stores. This substance is a potential hormone disrupter and harmful to human health.

Chapter five will prepare you to begin your transition to a whole food, plant-based lifestyle. This chapter includes guidance on reading food labels, eating out, travelling, and stocking your pantry, refrigerator, and freezer. In this chapter, you will find everything that you will need to begin leading a whole food, plant-based lifestyle. I explain how to make nut and seed milks and how to prepare and cook all your grains and beans, with added tips as you go. Superfoods and spices are also listed, and their benefits explained.

. . . plant proteins combined with complex carbohydrates are a much healthier alternative to animal-protein-based diets.

Chapter six contains over 200 vegan and gluten-free *Live Simply Plant Based* recipes, including feeding your body at the cellular level through liquid nutrition. You will also find specially formulated drinks to fuel post-exercise recovery, along with a section of many high-energy breakfast dishes to begin your day with proper nutrition. The main dishes are plant-protein rich and complex-carbohydrate dense, and ensure that you will receive all the nutrients your body needs to achieve and maintain great health. There is a section on dressings, toppings, and sauces, as well as one on healthy snacks.

The main dishes are plant-protein rich and carbohydrate dense, and ensure that you will receive all the nutrients your body needs

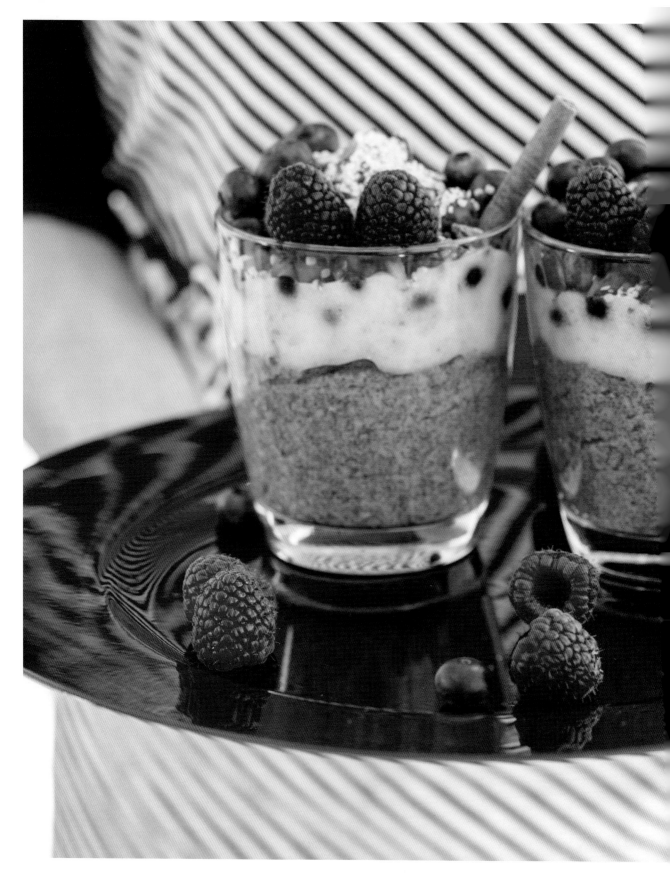

Part One

❧

The Plant-Based Lifestyle

Whether you want to throw yourself headlong into this lifestyle change or transition slowly over time, you will find many helpful tools and recipes in this book. Maybe you plan on preparing a plant-based meal a couple of days a week or just want to start eating a high-energy plant-based breakfast every day. Or maybe you are just interested in reading about all of the health benefits for now. Whatever it is that led you to purchase this book, I would like to personally thank you, and I hope you enjoy the read and the recipes!

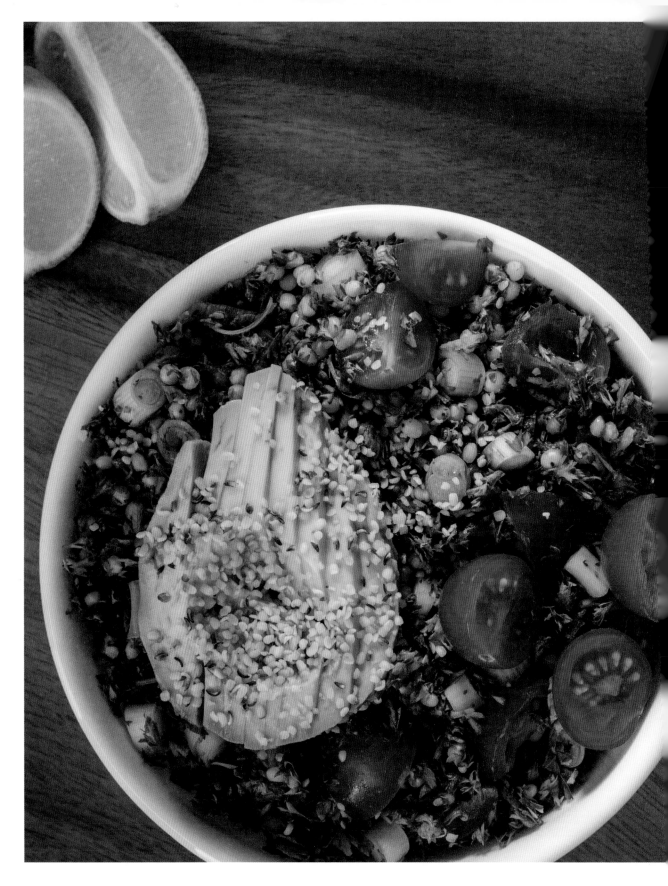

Understanding a Plant-Based Lifestyle

WHAT IS *LIVE SIMPLY PLANT-BASED?*

*L*ive Simply Plant-Based is not solely a diet, but a lifestyle. It is a lifestyle that is the healthiest for the long term, and the only potential downside is weight loss. That is a downside only if you do not wish to lose weight. I find myself eating all day long just to maintain my weight (which I don't really mind because I love to eat). So, if you love to eat and want to prevent or reverse disease, this is the lifestyle for you! It is made up of consuming plant-based whole foods, that is, eating plant foods as close to their natural state as possible with minimal processing. This includes all fruits, vegetables, whole grains, beans (legumes), nuts, and seeds. Incorporating this beneficial change into your life can have outstanding rewards. Not only will you see results quickly, but you will also look and feel great. You will have more energy, sleep better, and become sick less often.

I frequently see people over-exerting themselves in the gym and elsewhere through high impact, borderline dangerous workouts in an effort to burn extra calories to lose weight. These workouts that place too much stress on joints and muscles are not realistically maintainable over the long term by the majority of people.

What most people fail to realize is that the food they put into their body accounts for at least 70 percent of the way they look and

> *I find myself eating all day long just to maintain my weight (which I don't really mind because I love to eat).*

1

What most people fail to realize is that the food they put into their body accounts for at least 70 percent of the way they look and feel.

feel. If they made a lifestyle change to eating a whole food, plant-based diet, they could switch to lower impact workouts with less risk of over-stressing joints and muscles, thereby reducing the likelihood of injury. They could then lose the weight they desired and look and feel great! When we are young, a lot of us can get away with unhealthy eating behaviors, but this is temporary. Our metabolism begins to wane as we age, daily activity levels change, and improper diet can lead to diseases such as diabetes, heart disease, and cancer. Unfortunately, most of the time, only after the symptoms of disease begin do people start to make lifestyle changes. Keeping your body healthy from the inside out should begin as early as possible, but it is never too late to change.

A plant-based lifestyle will also help you to recover more quickly from exercise, have better mental clarity, and ward off unhealthy food cravings. Metabolism will begin to speed up, and body fat will be reduced. Whole plant foods are packed full of nutrients and they are low in calories and high in fiber, so they keep your furnace burning all day long. The fiber stabilizes blood sugar, and keeps you regular in the bathroom. Whole plant foods are easy on the digestive system and alkaline in nature, which keeps an unhealthy, acidic internal body environment at bay. When you feed your body with all the nutrients it needs, you will find that you have fewer cravings for unhealthy foods.

Plant foods have advantages over animal foods when it comes to digestibility. They contain many different enzymes allowing the body to digest efficiently. They also contain insoluble fiber that helps food move quickly through the digestive system, eliminating toxins along with it. On the other hand, animal products slow down digestion and elimination, thereby allowing toxins to remain stagnant in the body for long periods of time. This is extremely unhealthy! Consuming overly acidic foods is a major stressor of the immune system. Additionally, over-cooking foods, eating too fast, and overeating can stress the digestive system.

It is astonishing to me that despite the inadequacies of the omnivore diet plans such as Paleo, Atkins, and some other commercially promoted diet plans, they are still healthier than the standard American diet. The standard American diet is high in saturated fat and trans-fats, high in animal protein, low in fiber, highly processed, low in fruits and vegetables, and low in complex carbohydrates. Change is needed: people must begin to educate themselves on proper nutrition.

Although, some commercially promoted diet plans encourage plant food consumption, they frequently consist of a lot of packaged, nutritionally deficient, processed foods. Paleo and Atkins diets that promote high protein and low carbohydrate intake have been particularly controversial. People have claimed to lose weight and feel great on these diets. However, long-term use of these kinds of diet plans can be very dangerous. Increasing animal protein consumption equals an increase in saturated fat, and decreasing carbohydrates leads to a lower intake of fiber. This combination of increased saturated fat and lower intake of fiber elevates LDL (bad) cholesterol, lowers HDL (good) cholesterol, stresses the digestive system and kidneys, causes an acidic environment in the body, and can lead to insulin resistance.

The Paleo diet proposes that carbohydrates increase insulin, when, in reality, animal protein actually increases it more, as meat has the highest insulin response. In fact, animal fat causes almost the same insulin response as processed sugar.

Much research has been done on whole food, plant-based diets by pioneers in the fields of cardiology and nutrition, such as John A. McDougall, MD; Caldwell B. Esselstyn Jr., MD; T. Colin Campbell, PhD; and Dean Ornish, MD. Also, a study by Brie Turner-Mcgrievy showed significant evidence of the benefits of a vegan diet, when compared to vegetarians, pesco-vegetarians, semi-vegetarians, and omnivores—all diets focused on high-fiber and low-glycemic foods. Furthermore, the Turner-Mcgrievy study found that even though

. . . despite the inadequacies of the omnivore diet plans such as Paleo, Atkins, and some other commercially promoted diet plans, they are still healthier than the standard American diet.

semi-vegetarian and vegetarian diets are relatively healthy, vegans lost the most weight, while their antioxidant, folic acid, and potassium levels all increased. Additionally, there was no evidence of low calcium amongst the vegan group. All groups took B12 supplements, and vegans had the lowest saturated fat intake of just 7 percent. However, a vegan diet can be very unhealthy if it is composed of processed foods such as potato chips, soda, candy, and processed baked goods. When a vegan diet is followed as a whole food, plant-based diet, it is far superior to any other diet lifestyle.

A Whole Food, Plant-based lifestyle can:

- Boost metabolism
- Reduce body fat
- Reduce cholesterol
- Balance blood sugar
- Lower blood pressure
- Help build bone
- Prevent constipation
- Increase energy
- Reduce cravings
- Improve sleep
- Increase mental focus
- Speed recovery from exercise
- Improve overall health

DIABESITY AND A WHOLE FOOD, PLANT-BASED LIFESTYLE

Diabesity, the combination of obesity and diabetes, is a health condition caused by consuming detrimental, health-harming foods that is leading to a major epidemic in nations consuming a typical animal protein-based diet.

Michael Herschel Greger, MD, author and public health speaker on the benefits of a whole food, plant-based lifestyle explains very clearly the cause of Type 2 diabetes and insulin resistance. Glucose increases when a high fat diet is consumed. This in turn causes blood sugar levels to spike, which is the key to Type 2 diabetes. When we consume carbohydrates, our bodies break down starch into glucose so it can be used as the main energy source for our bodies. This glucose then needs insulin to access our muscle cells. Enzymes become activated to allow the glucose to enter muscle cells. If no insulin is available, glucose cannot access the muscle cells and remains in the blood. Additionally, insulin may not be available to allow glucose to enter the muscle cells to be used as energy, because of fat build-up in the muscle cells, which leads to insulin resistance. However, if we reduce the amount of fat we consume, insulin resistance disappears.

Insulin works most efficiently when a low-fat, plant-based diet is consumed. Therefore, high-fat, low-carbohydrate diets that claim to be healthy are false and dangerous. However, not all fats are created equal. The culprits of insulin resistance appear to be saturated fats which are found predominantly in animal products: meat, poultry, dairy, and eggs. Fats from plant sources such as nuts and seeds (with the exception of coconut oil) are mostly unsaturated, made up of polyunsaturated and monounsaturated fats, and these types of fats have beneficial effects on insulin resistance when used in moderation. One would think that the more weight we gain, the more fat cells we would accumulate. This however, is not the case. We are all born with the same number of fat cells, but our fat cells increase in size as we gain weight, and can shrink in size as we lose weight. When our fat cells keep increasing in size, they can spill over into the bloodstream and eventually lead to Type 2 diabetes. Fat also enters the blood stream from the food we consume. Even a slim person can have too much fat in his or her muscle cells from consuming a high-fat, low -carbohydrate diet.

The glycemic index is an important tool for those who need to control blood glucose levels, especially diabetics. David Jenkins, MD, invented the glycemic index, which ranks the rise in blood sugar following a meal. He began with a meal made up of 50 grams of white bread, which equals 100 percent on the glycemic index. The lower a food ranks on the index, the less its consumption causes a rise in blood sugar. Whole grains such as oats and bulgur wheat slow digestion because of their fiber content, and they do not cause a significant increase in blood sugar; therefore, they are ranked as low-glycemic foods.

For centuries, countries like Japan, India, and China consumed predominantly plant-based diets, and they had very low rates of diabetes. The low rate of diabetes makes perfect sense, as the fiber in whole plant-based foods ranks low on the glycemic index. On the other hand, now that these nations have moved away from the predominantly plant-based diet of high-fiber foods such as beans, their rates of diabetes have increased drastically. This trend has increased as they lower their consumption of whole plant-based foods but continue to consume increasing amounts of animal protein along with white rice, which has no or very little fiber and ranks high on the glycemic index. This trend is exacerbated by the fact that they are also now exposed to the Western diet of fast-food establishments.

Neal Barnard, MD, author and clinical researcher, conducted a very interesting study on patients with Type 2 diabetes. Ninety-nine individuals switched to a vegan diet after trying many different

For centuries, countries like Japan, India, and China consumed predominantly plant-based diets, and they had very low rates of diabetes.

diets without success. The vegan diet consisted of plant-based, low-glycemic index foods, with little or no oils. The results were amazing! Blood sugar levels dropped lower than they did with diabetes medications. The study participants lost weight slowly and naturally. Their cholesterol levels and blood pressure levels also dropped (very important to keep under control in diabetic patients). Eighteen months following the study, blood sugar levels remained under control and medications were reduced and some were even eliminated. The evidence of the benefits of a whole-food, plant-based diet in the prevention and even possible reversal of Type 2 diabetes is substantial. The seventh leading cause of death in the United States can be eliminated if we use whole plant-based foods as our medicine.

HEART DISEASE AND A WHOLE FOOD, PLANT-BASED LIFESTYLE

The benefits of a whole food, plant-based diet in combating heart disease have been well documented. Pioneers in the field of research such as Ornish and Esselstyn have proven in studies that a whole food, plant-based diet, when followed correctly, can prevent and even reverse cardiovascular disease. Ornish has accumulated a total of thirty-seven years of scientific research proving that beneficial changes in diet and lifestyle can significantly improve heart health.

Esselstyn contributed an article based on his research to the *Journal of Geriatric Cardiology*, "A Plant-based Diet and Coronary Artery Disease: A Mandate for Effective Therapy." I will just touch on the background of the article and treatment, however, if you would like to read the paper in full, please see the link below. In 1999 an autopsy study was performed on young adults in the US between the ages of seventeen and thirty-four years old who died from events unrelated to disease. The study showed that these young adults already had evidence of cardiovascular disease. Even though the cardiovascular disease was not severe enough to cause coronary events at the time of death, it most likely would have if they had lived longer. A similar finding of cardiovascular disease was discovered in young soldiers of the Korean War. During autopsy, 80 percent of soldiers with an average age of twenty were found to have cardiovascular disease. As a result of the findings in both the 1999 study and the Korean War soldier autopsy records, it was determined that the foundation for cardiovascular disease is established by the end of the high school years.

The conventional answer to this epidemic is a diet consisting of low-fat meat and dairy, exercise, and the use of prescription drugs. Unfortunately, even with these treatment options in place, cardiovascular disease still remains the number-one killer in the United States. In 1985, Esselstyn began a small study with twenty-four patients who suffered from severe cardiovascular disease. He placed them on a whole food, plant-based diet. During the years prior to the study, they had suffered, in total, forty-nine cardiovascular events, indicating that their disease was progressing. Eighteen of the original twenty-four patients continued with the program. After twelve years, twelve of the original twenty-four patients underwent follow-up angiograms. Four of the patients had not only halted, but significantly reversed, their cardiovascular disease. In 1994 a larger study was conducted with 198 patients. After four years, almost 95 percent of the patients who had stuck with the whole food, plant-based diet avoided any cardiovascular events, and of the twenty-one patients who had not stuck with the diet, 62 percent suffered heart-related events. I do want to point out that Esselstyn's whole food, plant-based diet consisted of no processed oils (including olive oil) at all in the diet.

Caldwell B Esselstyn, "A Plant-based Diet and Coronary Artery Disease: A Mandate for Effective Therapy," *Journal of Geriatric Cardiology*, 14:5 (2017): 317–320.

CANCER AND A WHOLE FOOD, PLANT-BASED LIFESTYLE

T. Colin Campbell, co-author of *The China Study* and well known for his studies on protein deficiency, has demonstrated through his studies that a healthy plant-based lifestyle can help to prevent, halt, and possibly even reverse cancer. His study on rats proved that a diet high in animal protein activates cancer, and the *China Study* proved that when people consumed whole food, plant-based diets in the regions of rural China, very little or no cancer was found there. In regions where people consumed diets high in animal protein, a high rate of all forms of cancer was found. Cancer is the number-two killer of men and women in the United States.

The pharmaceutical approach to cancer treatment focuses on using a single extracted chemical to target a specific type of cancer. Obviously, this is not working. Cancer is still our number-two killer. Billions of dollars have been wasted on cancer drugs in the US, and millions of lives have been lost in the process; when all we needed to do is look at what we feed our bodies. We know that when people migrate from one country to another (an example of this would be Japanese people migrating to the United States), and then begin consuming the typical Western diet, they begin to get the typical Western diseases. So genetics may not play as big a part in cancer formation as previously thought.

Campbell has conducted many studies proving that a diet high in animal protein is a breeding ground for cancer. Whole foods come from nature. Regardless of your blood type or uniqueness, everyone can thrive on a whole food, plant-based diet. There is no downside to eating this way, and nutrient intake increases. We do not need a high-animal-protein diet to be healthy. We can get all the protein that we require from plants, and plant foods have many nutritional properties that perform different functions within the body. Whole foods are the best way for the body to

In regions where people consumed diets high in animal protein, a high rate of all forms of cancer was found.

receive nutrition, and supplements should not be used to take the place of a whole food, plant-based diet. Nutrients from consuming the whole food are far superior to nutrients isolated into supplement form.

Nature has already provided us with the diet our body requires, so why would we eat any differently? Especially when we know that it can make us sick! When people switch to a whole food, plant-based lifestyle, after just one week they can have dramatic changes in their health. Just imagine what it can do for health over the long term. Plants have the power to heal, and excessive dairy and meat consumption is a danger to human health. It increases the risk of diabesity, heart disease, and cancer, along with many other diseases.

Nature has already provided us with the diet our body requires, so why would we eat any differently?

Plant-Based Vegan Stories

Since becoming focused on the benefits of a whole food, plant-based lifestyle, I have encountered a number of individuals who have shared with me their personal experiences. These experiences demonstrate the successful resolution of health issues as a result of transforming to a whole food, plant-based diet. Below are a few of the stories individuals have shared with me. I am including them in this book, as nothing demonstrates success as vividly as personal experiences of people who have taken it upon themselves to make proper nourishment of their bodies a priority to Live!

Shane P.

"Descending from a family of high blood pressure and heart disease should have been all the motivation I needed to get my own health sorted, but being only twenty-six years old, I thought I was invincible.

Cholesterol of 7.8 and 12 kg (over 26 lb.) overweight, with my first child on the way, was where it all started to click.

"Cutting out fatty foods and lowering sugar intake was the first step, which saw my LDL and HDL readings change dramatically and my weight came down 7 kg (over 15 lb.) over the next few years, but both plateaued no matter what I did or how hard I tried.

"I thought running 40–50 kilometers (25–30 miles) per week and what I though was "clean eating" was all that was required, until colleagues began constantly drumming "Vegan, vegan, vegan" into my head for months. One day I cracked and went cold-turkey, full vegan.

"The first weeks were the hardest, but over the next six months I saw awesome results, which gave me a whole new burst of life, my energy level and my mind were on a whole new level.

"Cholesterol down to 4.8 (and still falling), sitting pretty at 75 kg (165 lb.), and I completed my first 42-km (26-mile) marathon in sub-four hours.

"I love cheese and wine nights and BBQs with family and friends, but enjoying a long, healthy life with my kids is a lot higher on my list."

Dale A.

"My story begins when I was at work (I work two weeks on, one week off). We were encouraged to participate in a mini health screen; this included glucose levels, blood pressure checks, etc. I only joined in at the last minute, as I exercised a lot and considered myself quite fit and am also a non-smoker.

"So, it came as a surprise to me that I recorded a high blood-pressure reading and was advised to go and see the site medic to confirm that it wasn't just a one-off event. So off I went and had it checked by the medic and, yes, still high, so he advised me to book an appointment with my local doctor for when I got home on R &

R. While I was waiting for my work swing to finish, I visited the medic once per shift and wrote down my blood pressure readings to pass on to the doctor.

"So off to the doctors I went and, sure enough, I still had high blood pressure, so he then made me go and get some blood tests done, and the end result was I was also on the borderline of having Type 2 diabetes as well as having a high cholesterol level, a bit of a shock to say the least.

"He then said I had two choices: I could either start taking medication for my ailments immediately or I could review and change my lifestyle and eating habits.

"A stroke of luck for me was that I had only just finished reading *The China Study* book by T. Colin Campbell. So, armed with this knowledge, my response was I would change my lifestyle and eating habits, as the thought of taking medication for the rest of my life was very unappealing.

"So, I then started living according to *The China Study* as best I could. If I had to put a percentage to that, I would say about 70 percent. When you work away, you can tend to be at the mercy of what type of food is available and how it is prepared, so you try to do as best you can. I also had to get my blood work checked every six months to start with, and each time my results improved, so after three visits since the initial test my results had plummeted back to very good levels. I now only get my blood tests done annually just to keep track. As an added bonus of eating well I also lost 12 kg (over 26 lb.).

"I have to say, I was fortunate that my doctor has also read *The China Study* and was very supportive of my tackling my ailments through good nutrition."

Andrew P.

"My story so far:

"For most of my life I have been overweight. It's the usual story of overeating and drinking too much alcohol. My diet was terrible: meats, starchy foods, takeaways, and beers, sometimes the occasional veggie or fruit. Although I knew I was overweight, I did not really consider myself to be obese, but I was. At 179 cm (around 5'9") and 94 kg (almost 207 lb.), it put me into the obese category, which was having an impact on both my physical and mental health. There are two aliments which currently trouble me: the first one is prostate cancer and the other is an irregular heartbeat, which occurs randomly. It's more miss a beat than irregular, but it has hospitalized me in the past. The heart problem started in 2001 and I've learnt to live with it. Not life threatening but I become concerned when it starts playing up.

"The cancer was discovered in November 2015. I went for my annual blood tests the September of that year, and the results came back with an elevated PSA reading. My GP referred me to a urology specialist, who booked me in for a biopsy. It was then discovered that I had two tumors, one measuring 3 mm and the other 0.3 mm, in the prostate. Not the sort of joyful news I was hoping for.

"Prior to the discovery of the prostate cancer, I had been reading Colin T Campbell's book, as suggested by Dale to help with the heart problem. I was so glad that I had taken Dale's advice and read the book. It helped me to understand what was happening to my body and why. It explained to me how the foods that we eat are major contributors to our health and how poor food choices lead to poor health. So, I began the dietary change that I needed to help with my aliments.

"I was able to reduce my PSA level from 5.2 to 3.1 within a few months on a vegan diet. The specialist I am seeing was happy and suggested an annual review. He did not foresee any immediate danger of the cancer's growing since my levels had dropped.

"The diet has also given me extra energy, and I now visit the gym on a regular basis.

"Timeline:

- **Sept 2015,** discovered that I had a PSA level of 5.2
- **Nov 2015,** PSA level had dropped to 4.1 by the time I had the biopsy
- **Nov 2015,** biopsy results showed two tumors; one 3 mm the other 0.3 mm
- **Dec 2015,** PSA level continued to drop to 3.1
- **April 2016,** had a MRI scan, results were negative—no tumors found
- **Oct 2016,** PSA level remaining at 3.1
- **Oct 2017,** PSA level raised to 4.1. I had begun eating animal products earlier this year, small quantities but enough to cause a rise in the PSA level. Back on full vegan diet again as of now."
- **Nov 2017,** PSA dropped to 3.1
- **Feb 2018,** results from 2nd biopsy were negative, cancer- and tumor-free. Even the tumors from the 1st biopsy have disappeared. I can now say with confidence that this is a result of my vegan diet.

STRESS-REDUCING PRACTICES

Stress affects all of us. Our environment adds stress to our lives on a daily basis, pushing the body into a state of overstimulation. Many people are not even aware of how their daily living habits are affecting their health: physically, emotionally, physiologically, and psychologically. What we put into our bodies, what we deal with at work, air pollutants, unhealthy relationships, and time constraints all add extreme pressure. However, when stress is utilized in a positive way, it can serve us well. Exercise is stress placed upon the body that can be very beneficial. Moderate exercise followed by rest for recovery serves the body and the mind well, but when the body is repeatedly pushed beyond its capability and not enough time allotted to rest, the body is unable to recover properly, and physical and mental symptoms soon begin to manifest. Lack of exercise also adds unhealthy stress, muscles become weak, body fat increases, mental clarity begins to wane, and joints begin to deteriorate.

The two main stress hormones that the body manufactures are DHEA and cortisol. These hormones are produced in the adrenal glands, which are located on top of the kidneys. When the body is stressed it goes into a fight-or-flight response. This response can be very positive when it is warranted, as in the need to run from a dangerous situation. The fight-or-flight response causes cortisol levels to rise, reflexes and senses to quicken, giving the body the energy to run. However, when unwelcome stress causes us to be in a constant state of fight or flight, we can eventually end up with adrenal fatigue and cortisol hormones that can no longer function optimally. This can lead to conditions such as chronic fatigue, fibromyalgia, anxiety disorder, and many more. DHEA is a powerful anti-aging hormone, and low levels of DHEA are found among people suffering with depression, cognitive decline, and other neurological disorders. Balance of cortisol and DHEA is vital to a healthy bodily system. What we put into our bodies is the number-one stressor that we have total control over. When we begin a healthy regime from the inside out, other healthy rituals such as meditation and exercise tend to follow.

MEDITATION

Meditation is an anti-aging tool that can also ward off depression and anxiety.

One of the most important stress-reducing practices is taking time out for yourself at least once a day, even if it is only for ten minutes to just sit and relax in comfortable, safe space. Close your eyes and bring your attention to your breath, just observing your body along with your breath. Set a timer, starting with five minutes, and see if you can increase to fifteen or even thirty minutes over time. Meditation increases self-awareness, which in turn allows you to be in synch with your body, because it cleans and cleanses the mind and reduces stress, meditation is an anti-aging tool that can also ward off depression and anxiety. In addition to allowing you to be more accepting of yourself and of others, meditation helps you to stay present and enjoy the moment. It is amazing what this little ritual can do for your whole well-being.

LOW-IMPACT EXERCISE

Walking, swimming, and gentle yoga, are all great forms of low-impact movement to get the body in motion. Taking a brisk walk for just thirty minutes a day can have great benefits for your health. Walking boosts metabolism, helps to build bone, lowers blood pressure, and improves mood. Swimming provides a complete body workout and builds endurance and strength. Swimming also strengthens the heart and lungs and tones muscles. Yoga improves flexibility and balance, tones and strengthens muscles, improves respiration and self-awareness, calms stress and anxiety, improves posture, and boosts immunity.

WEIGHT TRAINING

Using light weights and slowing down and increasing the number of repetitions performed can be just as beneficial in increasing muscle size and strength as lifting heavy weights to failure. Lifting lighter weights also reduces the risk of injury and places less stress on the joints. Weight training is bone-building, metabolism-boosting, and body-shaping. If you are unsure how to lift weights correctly, hire a certified personal trainer for a few sessions. Let him or her know before you begin that you would like to lift light weights slowly with higher repetitions to build strength and muscle. Tell him or her that you would like to focus on form and technique. Once you have learned the correct technique, you can then train independently.

There are many different forms of stress-reducing practices and exercise activities to take part in, but I have chosen these particular forms of exercise because they can be performed by everyone regardless of age and physical fitness level.

NUTRITION AND EXERCISE

Proper nutrition is vital to exercise. Fueling your body with the right foods before and after working out can make all the difference to beneficial gains and recovery. All my recipes in this book are aimed at fueling the body with nutrient-dense foods to constantly supply the cells with energy. It is pointless to work out in the gym only to reward yourself with an ice-cream smoothie or burger and fries afterward. These foods not only drain the body of

Fueling your body with the right foods before and after working out can make all the difference to beneficial gains and recovery.

vital nutrients, they are heavy, harmful, and detrimental to exercise recovery. It would be like taking three steps forward and fifteen steps back. Supplying your body with whole, plant-based foods on a regular basis will keep your body light and well fueled for working out regularly.

A great post-workout recovery would be a *Live* liquid nutrition recovery drink, consumed within forty-five minutes of working out. All these drinks are high in fruit, therefore, high in carbohydrates, and contain a lower amount of plant protein, a perfect balance for exercise recovery. It is a mistake to restrict calorie consumption following exercise, especially if your energy reserves are low. Blood sugar may start to drop and fatigue will set in if energy needs are not met with food. Also, it will slow recovery and hinder progress. An hour or so following your post-workout snack you can enjoy a *Live Simply Plant-Based* main dish that is higher in protein and fiber.

The High Protein and Low Carbohydrate Myths

THE HIGH PROTEIN MYTH

The high protein myth is the proposition that you need to consume large quantities of animal proteins (meat, dairy, poultry, eggs, whey protein powders, egg white protein powders, etc.) to maintain and build muscle mass and recover and repair muscles following intense workouts.

The human body's minimum requirement for adequate daily protein intake is between 8 and 12 percent of total daily calorie intake. Pregnant women (for the development of the develop-ing fetus) and elite athletes (to maintain lean muscle mass, and to facilitate muscle recovery and repair) should aim for a minimum of 12 percent, and the average person should be closer to a mini-mum of 8 percent protein from daily calorie intake. We can easily achieve these requirements while following a *Live Simply Plant-based Lifestyle*. Fruits, vegetables, whole grains, legumes, nuts, and seeds all contain protein. Whole grains, legumes, nuts, and seeds contain the highest amount of protein in the plant kingdom. Many elite athletes have proven that it is possible to thrive and win without the consumption of animal protein. In fact, athletes are at a greater advantage when consuming whole plant foods, as animal protein is acidic in nature, stresses the liver and kidneys, and causes inflammation throughout the body. Furthermore,

Fruits, vegetables, whole grains, legumes, nuts, and seeds all contain protein.

animal protein slows down digestion and, when over–consumed, can lead to constipation.

Plant protein on the other hand, is nutrient dense, calorie light, alkaline, anti-inflammatory in nature, aids in digestion, and keeps the bowels regular. The powerful antioxidant, anti-inflammatory nutrients found in plant foods allow the body to recover more quickly from injury and high-intensity workouts, and help increase energy levels. Plants do not contain the growth hormones, antibiotics, and highly saturated fats that are contained in animal proteins.

The high protein myth that consumption of large quantities of animal protein is necessary to achieve strength and vitality, whether from eating meat or filling up on whey protein shakes, should be laid to rest as more and more people are realizing the multitude of benefits of consuming lower levels of protein through the intake of whole plant foods.

Let's take a look at the belief that if you are vegan, then you are probably protein deficient. This would only be true if you were a very unhealthy vegan. It is virtually impossible to be protein deficient if you are consuming a healthy, varied vegan diet that includes whole fruits, vegetables, grains, legumes, nuts, and seeds. The reason some people lose too much weight when switching to a whole food, plant-based lifestyle is not from protein deficiency, but from not consuming enough calories.

Whole plant foods are relatively low in calories, with the exception of nuts, seeds, and dried fruit. Therefore, it is necessary to eat more plant foods to sustain calorie needs and, thereby, maintain weight. Adding more grains, legumes, nuts, and seeds along with your fruits and vegetables will help increase calorie consumption. If you are looking to lose weight, you may want to cut back on your calorie intake. Another advantage of eating whole plant foods is that the fiber content of plant foods fills you up, keeps your blood sugar stable, and helps to ward off unhealthy food cravings.

It is virtually impossible to be protein deficient if you are consuming a healthy, varied vegan diet . . .

Absent a medical condition, it would be virtually impossible to be obese on a whole foods, plant-based diet.

In addition to the high protein myth, another fallacy is that plant proteins are not complete proteins. Some plant proteins are complete proteins, and complete proteins are made up of the eight essential amino acids, which are found abundantly in the plant kingdom. Some examples of complete plant proteins are: amaranth, soy, quinoa, buckwheat, chia, hemp, chlorella or spirulina with whole grains or nuts, wholegrain rice with beans, hummus with pita, and nut butter with whole grain bread.

Let's take a closer look at these plant proteins and the eight essential amino acids.

. . . another fallacy is that plant proteins are not complete proteins.

PLANTS CONTAINING THE HIGHEST AMOUNTS OF PROTEIN

- **Legumes**: Primarily known as beans or pulses, not only consists of beans and peas, but also includes alfalfa, tamarind, peanuts, carob, mesquite, and clover. Highest sources of protein:

    - **Beans** ~ Includes all beans (white, red, fava, mung, soy, anasazi, pinto, kidney, black, navy, garbanzo, lima, and black-eyed peas) ~ The average source of protein content for cooked beans is around 15 g per cup, with soybeans having the highest protein content of almost 29 g per cup. Soybeans provide a good source of all eight essential amino acids.

    - **Peas and lentils** ~ Includes chana dahl, dahl, french lentils, green lentils, red lentils, green split peas, and yellow split peas. Cooked lentils average around 18 g of protein, and split peas around 16 g of protein per cup.

 ✎ **Peanuts** ~ Pack a punch in the legume protein department with 25 g per cup.

❀ **Whole Grains**: Include brown, red, and black rice, quinoa, millet, amaranth, buckwheat, barley, bulgur, oats, whole wheat, spelt, kamut, rye, and teff. Highest sources of protein:

 ✎ **Spelt** ~ An ancient grain, mild and easily digested. It hasn't been altered in any way and therefore does not generally cause gluten sensitivity. Cooked, it contains around 11 g of protein per cup.

 ✎ **Amaranth** ~ A slightly finer grain than quinoa and a great addition to many foods. Sticky when cooked. It can be eaten for breakfast or as a side dish mixed with vegetables. Cooked, it contains a little over 9 g of protein per cup.

 ✎ **Quinoa** ~ More of a seed than a grain, cooks just like a grain and can be used in place of rice. High in nutrition with a slight nutty flavor. Cooked, it contains almost 9 g of protein per cup.

❀ **Nuts**: Includes almonds, Brazils, cashews, chestnuts, hazelnuts, macadamias, pecans, pine nuts, pistachios, and walnuts.

 ✎ **Pistachios** ~ Rank the highest in protein with around 25 g of protein per cup.

- ⟋ **Almonds** ~ Contain around 21 g of protein per cup.

◉ **Seeds**: Includes flax, sunflower, pumpkin, sesame, hemp, and chia.

- ⟋ **Hemp seeds** ~ Contain the highest amount of protein per cup, with over 30 g.

- ⟋ **Pumpkin seeds** ~ Contain around 28 g of protein per cup.

◀ However, a cup is not a serving size as nuts are high in fat, so a serving size would generally be about ¼ to ⅓ cup.

◀ Again, a cup is not a serving size when it comes to seeds. A generous serving size would be ¼ to ⅓ cup.

THE EIGHT ESSENTIAL AMINO ACIDS

◉ **Leucine** • Also known as BCAA (branched chain amino acid), stimulates muscle growth and strength, aids in the stabilization of blood sugar levels, and enhances mood, warding off depression. Plants containing a good source of leucine are: leafy greens, seaweed, whole grains, peas, soy, sunflower seeds, figs, avocados, bananas, dates, apples, pears, blueberries, whole grain rice, and olives.

◉ **Isoleucine** • Also a BCAA and very closely related to leucine, but with different functions. It increases energy production by being broken down within muscle tissue. Plants containing a good source of isoleucine are: soy, lentils, brown rice, beans, almonds, oats, hemp seeds, chia seeds, pumpkin seeds, sunflower seeds, sesame seeds, quinoa, apples, kiwis, blueberries, apricots, peaches, and cranberries

❀ **Lysine** ~ Plays a big part in the absorption of calcium, helps the body to recover from injury and surgery, and aids in the production of enzymes and hormones. Plants containing a good source of lysine are: watercress, seaweed, amaranth, soybeans, navy beans, kidney beans, split peas, lentils, chickpeas, spirulina, and chlorella.

❀ **Methionine** ~ Promotes the growth of new blood vessels. Plants containing a good source of methionine are: seaweed, Brazil nuts, sesame seeds, soy, wheat germ, oats, peanuts, chickpeas, corn, almonds, pinto beans, lentils, whole grain rice, grapes, and oranges.

❀ **Phenylalanine** ~ Converts to tyrosine following digestion and manufactures thyroid hormones, proteins, and brain chemicals. Babies are screened at birth for PKU (Phenylketonuria), a rare genetic disease that causes a buildup of phenylalanine in the body, which can result in irreversible brain damage. Plants containing a good source of phenylalanine are: soy, spirulina, seaweed, pumpkin seeds, figs, beans, lentils, whole grains, raisins, avocados, and olives.

❀ **Threonine** ~ Increases immune function and aids in the biosynthesis of proteins, stimulating growth and recovery of muscle tissue. Plants containing a good source of threonine are: watercress, spirulina, chlorella, leafy greens, chia seeds, hemp seeds, soybeans, pumpkin, sprouted grains, almonds, quinoa, wheat, figs, sesame seeds, and avocados.

❀ **Tryptophan** ~ A neurotransmitter, calming to the
nervous system, aids in restful sleep and assists in
muscle repair and growth. Plants containing good
sources of tryptophan are: oats, oat bran, soy,
pumpkin and squash seeds, beans, lentils, sweet
potatoes, beets, parsley, hemp seeds, chia seeds,
leafy greens, lettuce, Chinese cabbage, chives,
cauliflower, mushrooms, asparagus, kale, broccoli,
brussel sprouts, tomatoes, and carrots.

❀ **Valine** ~ Also a BCAA, is important in the
regulation of blood sugar, providing extra glucose
during exercise, and also assists in the normal
growth and repair of muscle tissue. Plants
containing good sources of valine are: soy, pumpkin
seeds, pistachios, sunflower seeds, chia seeds,
almonds, beans, lentils, mushrooms, and whole
grains.

As detailed in this section you can see that all eight essential amino
acids are abundant in the plant kingdom, and by consuming a variety of whole plant foods it is possible to easily obtain all of them
from plants alone.

ACID REFLUX AND HIGH-PROTEIN DIETS

One of the most commonly diagnosed diseases in the United
States is gastroesophageal reflux disease (GERD); more than three
million people are diagnosed every year. GERD is a condition in
which stomach acid flows up into the esophagus on a regular
basis, causing a range of symptoms such as heartburn, nausea,
vomiting, fullness in the stomach, gnawing stomach pain, a feeling

of a lump in the throat, sore throat, and possibly even asthma. The most commonly prescribed form of treatment is proton pump inhibitors, such as Prilosec and Nexium. It amazes me that people are willing to take a drug and continue with their regular dietary eating habits, when all that is needed in most cases to eliminate this condition is a dietary lifestyle change. High-animal-protein diets are not only high in fat, but also very acid-forming in the body. All animal proteins are acidic in nature, causing an imbalance in pH and a reduction in good bacteria.

Plants are alkaline in nature and easily digested. I know many individuals who previously suffered tremendously from GERD, and after switching to a whole food, plant-based diet, saw their symptoms disappear. I am one of those individuals. For suffers of GERD, an endoscopy is the most commonly overprescribed invasive procedure performed today, when simple dietary changes should be the first line of treatment.

All animal proteins are acidic in nature, causing an imbalance in pH and a reduction in good bacteria.

LACTOSE INTOLERANCE AND CASEIN SENSITIVITY

Lactose intolerance is the inability to completely digest the milk sugar known as lactose. This condition is caused by an insufficiency of the enzyme lactase, which is made in the small intestine. Lactase separates lactose into glucose and galactose. A person with lactose intolerance is unable to digest all of the lactose in milk and/or milk products, which can result in indigestion, gas, diarrhea, bloating, inflammation, and abdominal cramps. The condition can vary from person to person. One in four infants is lactose intolerant, along with up to 75 percent of the world's population. Milk is served regularly in schools, and children suffer with mild to moderate symptoms on a daily basis. Children who are frequent milk consumers also suffer with recurrent ear infections and/or sinus related symptoms, and adults with lactose intolerance tend to continue to consume milk throughout their lives even though they suffer digestive upsets.

The protein casein, found in milk, is a common food allergen, and symptoms from consuming casein can range from mild to severe. Symptoms of casein sensitivity include mild indigestion to severe gastrointestinal problems. Cow's milk is produced to nourish baby cows. A baby cow grows from around sixty pounds at birth to a whopping four hundred pounds in adulthood. If cow's milk were made for human consumption, why would baby formula have to be altered to mimic human breast milk? Also, why would the majority of the world's population be lactose intolerant? This proves that humans were not meant to consume cow's milk. Cow's milk is detrimental to human health!

Further proof of the harmful effects of cow's milk was discovered by T. Colin Campbell, who is well known for the *China Study*. Campbell conducted an experimental study of rats that linked cancerous tumor formation to casein, the protein found in cow's milk. The study methodology involved injecting the rats with the carcinogen aflatoxin, and then feeding the rats casein. The results were astonishing. Campbell found that he could turn cancer on and off by increasing and decreasing the amount of casein fed to the rats. When the rats were fed a diet of 20 percent casein, they all grew cancerous tumors, but when he reduced their intake to 5 percent, the tumors disappeared. Campbell also tried feeding the rats plant protein, and regardless of the amount of plant protein he fed to the rats, tumors did not form.

CALCIUM AND A PLANT-BASED LIFESTYLE

If you are concerned about obtaining enough calcium from consuming a whole food, plant-based diet, you should not be as there are many plant foods rich in calcium.

Plant foods high in calcium:

- Dark green leafy vegetables
- Soybeans and soy products, e.g., tofu
- Almonds
- Broccoli
- Cabbage
- Butternut squash
- Sweet potatoes
- Celery
- Beans
- Carrots
- Sesame seeds
- Chia seeds
- Hemp seeds
- Amaranth
- Oranges
- Figs
- Blackberries

I am sure I have left out many more plant foods rich in calcium, but, as you can see from this list, there is no reason to believe that we need dairy products to obtain sufficient levels of calcium in the diet. These calcium-rich plant foods are also packed full of many other nutritional benefits, making them much better choices.

THE LOW CARBOHYDRATE MYTH

The low carbohydrate myth usually goes hand in hand with the high protein myth. So many high-protein, low-carbohydrate diets have come and gone. These diets are not sustainable long term because of their negative health effects.

Not all carbohydrates are created equal. Simple carbohydrates, which include foods such as white pasta, white rice, sugar, and many other processed foods, are nutrient deficient and lack fiber. Complex carbohydrates, which include whole grains, beans, and vegetables, are nutrient dense and loaded with fiber. Although fruits are complex in nature and extremely nutrient dense, they actually work more like simple carbohydrates by boosting energy levels rapidly and increasing blood sugar.

Taking complex carbohydrates out of the diet or reducing intake drastically can have very negative consequences on overall health, and can lead to fatigue and lack of mental clarity. Complex carbohydrates supply the body with long-lasting energy and help to keep the mind alert and focused, so it is important to include complex carbohydrates at every meal. Complex carbohydrates are the main source of calories/energy in a healthy diet.

Low-carbohydrate diets are touted to lower insulin levels, which may be true if the carbohydrates being reduced are simple carbohydrates coming from processed foods. However, when complex carbohydrates are lowered significantly, and the diet is high in animal protein, insulin levels will rise rather than fall. Animal protein has a higher insulin response than almost all car-bohydrates, with the exception of simple sugar, which is nearly equivalent to animal protein in insulin response. Animal protein contains fat, and fat is readily stored in the body without much effort. However, converting consumed carbohydrates to fat is very costly to the body, burning up to ten times as many calories as

Complex carbohydrates are the main source of calories/energy in a healthy diet.

storing consumed animal fats. Simple carbohydrates raise insulin levels and, when consumed along with animal fat as they so often are, can eventually lead to diabetes and obesity, diabesity.

A diet high in animal protein is also a diet high in saturated fat. Known as a ketogenic diet, this type of high-animal-protein/high-saturated-fat diet leads to insulin resistance. When too much saturated fat enters the muscle cells it blocks the entry of glucose to the muscle cells. Insulin is the key factor to allowing glucose to enter, but when fat is blocking the entrance to the muscle cells, insulin cannot work and glucose has nowhere to go, so it remains in the bloodstream. When animal protein/saturated fat is reduced, insulin resistance disappears and glucose is allowed to enter the muscle cells to be used as energy. When a diet rich in saturated fat was compared to a diet rich in carbohydrates, the high-fat diet increased blood sugar levels twice as much as the high-carbohydrate diet.

. . . the high-fat diet increased blood sugar levels twice as much as the high-carbohydrate diet.

WHAT IS A COMPLEX CARBOHYDRATE?

A complex carbohydrate is referred to as complex because it is made up of many sugar molecules strung together like a necklace. Complex carbohydrates are also full of fiber, making them an excellent source of fulfillment. They are also high in vitamins and minerals, assisting the body in promoting good health. Complex carbohydrates are found in abundance in the plant kingdom. Excellent sources of complex carbohydrates include all whole grains, beans, and vegetables. Although fruit is considered a simple carbohydrate, it is still an important food in a healthy diet due to its abundance of nutrients, and it is an excellent source of quick and easily digestible energy.

WHAT IS A SIMPLE CARBOHYDRATE?

A simple carbohydrate is referred to as simple because it is made up of just one or two sugar molecules. With the exception of fruit, most simple carbohydrates should be avoided, as they are stripped of their fiber and lack nutrients. Sources of simple carbohydrates to be avoided include sugar, white pasta, white bread, white rice, white flour, candy, and all sugary processed and baked foods.

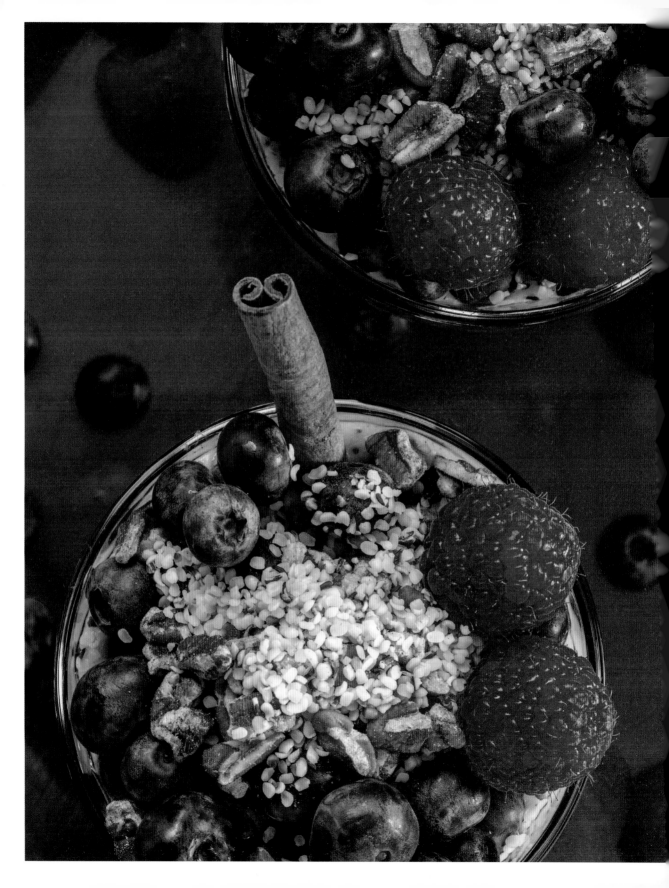

Acid/Alkaline Balance

The pH scale (potential of hydrogen) is a measure of the acidity or alkalinity of water soluble substances. Values on the pH scale runs from 1 to 14. The number 7 indicates neutral (neither acid nor alkaline), and any number below 7 indicates acidity, with number 1 being the most acidic. Numbers above 7 indicate alkalinity, with number 14 being the most alkaline. The human body is an amazing machine that has the capability to balance pH levels, but when we constantly bombard our bodies with acid-forming foods, as is typical when eating the standard American diet, the body begins to show signs of inflammation and disease. It is vital to consume the foods necessary to assist the body in maintaining homeostasis. The more alkaline foods we consume, the healthier the body becomes. The standard American diet is acidic in nature, because it is high in animal protein and processed foods which are acid-forming within body.

The more alkaline foods we consume, the healthier the body becomes.

A whole food, plant-based diet is naturally alkaline in nature because the majority of plants are alkaline-forming. The human body has the ability to balance pH levels to a certain extent. However, when the body is overloaded day after day, for long periods of time, with acid-forming foods such as animal proteins, the immune system starts to falter, making the body more susceptible to illness. An example of this is acid reflux disease.

An acidic bodily environment increases inflammation, and can also increase the risk of kidney stones. It can lead to arthritic conditions, encourage bone loss, and can also stress the adrenal glands, which can lead to chronic fatigue and waning mental focus. Low grade acidosis (when the body is in a constant acidic state) is a breeding ground for viruses, parasites, and unhealthy bacteria, which weakens the immune system even further.

Alkaline-forming foods are vital to health, and chlorophyll-rich plant foods are highly alkaline. They clean and cleanse the body, helping to keep an alkaline internal environment, and an optimally functioning body. Plants increase energy levels, help balance cortisol, and promote mental alertness. For the body's pH level to be balanced, the diet should consist of at least 75 percent alkaline foods. However, you do not need to be too concerned about consuming the correct percentage of alkaline foods every day if you are following a *Live Simply Plant-Based* lifestyle. This lifestyle fosters consumption of a diet consisting mostly of highly alkaline plant foods. Combining slightly acidic plant foods with mostly highly alkaline plants helps to neutralize acidity, thereby supporting a healthy bodily environment. By eating this way, you will also receive all the nutrients your body needs for high energy to enjoy a full and active life. Just remember to take time for yourself, to meditate or sit quietly, and also take part in your favorite exercise activities to help calm the body and mind. This will help reduce stress and anxiety, which can also significantly affect acid/alkaline balance.

Alkaline-forming foods are much easier on the digestive system, working with the body instead of against it. Acid-forming foods work against the body, slowing down digestion, taxing the liver and kidneys, and congesting the colon. Alkaline foods are nutrient and water dense, they move efficiently through the digestive system, cleaning and cleansing the liver and kidneys, and sweeping the colon clean. Here is a list of some alkaline-forming and acid-forming foods. Even though citrus fruits rank low on the pH scale, once digested

Plants increase energy levels, help balance cortisol, and promote mental alertness.

they actually become alkaline. As you can see from the following lists, almost all fruits and vegetables are alkaline, and all animal products are acid-producing.

Alkaline and Acid-Forming Foods

Alkaline Foods

Plant proteins

Almonds
Amaranth
Black rice
Brazil nuts
Cashews
Chestnuts
Flaxseeds
Hazelnuts
Hemp seeds
Chia seeds
Kamut
Pine nuts
Pumpkin seeds
Quinoa
Rye
Sesame seeds
Spelt
Teff
Wild rice

Grains

Amaranth
Black Rice
Kamut
Millet
Quinoa
Rye
Sorghum
Spelt
Teff
Wild rice
Red rice
Buckwheat

Vegetables

Avocado
Arugula
Bell peppers
Broccoli
Cabbage
Celery
Chard
Cilantro
Cucumber
Dandelion greens
Green beans
Leeks
Peas
Garbanzo beans
Kale
Lettuce
Mushrooms
Okra
Olives (and olive oil)
Onions
Parsley
Sea vegetables
    (wakame, dulse,
    arame, hijiki, nori)
Squash
Sweet potatoes
Tomatoes–cherry
    and plum only
Turnip greens
Watercress
Yams
Zucchini

Fruits

Apples
Avocados
Bananas
Berries
Cantaloupe
Cherries
Coconut
Currants
Dates
Elderberries
Figs
Grapes
Grapefruit
Lemons
Limes
Mango
Melons
Nectarines
Oranges
Papayas
Peaches
Pears
Pineapple
Plums
Pomegranates
Prunes
Raisins

Herbs and Spices

Basil
Bay leaf
Cayenne
Chili pepper
Cilantro
Coriander
Cumin

Alkaline and Acid Forming Foods

Alkaline Foods (continued)

Curry
Dill
Ginger
Marjoram
Onion powder
Oregano
Sesame/Seaweed
  Gomasio
Himalayan pink
  sea salt

Sage
Sweet basil
Tarragon
Thyme

Condiments

Apple cider vinegar
Balsamic vinegar

Neutral

Coconut
Macadamia
Coconut nectar
Agave nectar
Brazil nuts
Cashews

Slightly Acidic

Beans
Chickpeas
Lentils
Oats
Sunflower seeds
Brown rice
Walnuts
Pecans
Pistachios

Very Acidic

Animal Proteins

Beef
Chicken
Dairy
Eggs
Fish
Lamb
Pork
Shellfish
Turkey
Veal
Venison
Whey

Grains

Barley
Bran (oat, wheat)
Corn
Flour (wheat, white)
White rice
Wheat

Dairy

Butter
Cheese
Ice cream
Milk

Fruit

Cranberries

Drinks

Beer
Coffee
Juices (processed)
Liquor
Soda

Additional

Artificial sweeteners
White sugar
Processed breakfast
  cereals
Candy
Prescription drugs
Synthetic
  multivitamins
peanuts

Note: All herbs and spices
are alkaline or neutral.

Dangers of GMOs, Excitotoxins, and BPA

GMOS (GENETICALLY MODIFIED ORGANISMS)

Most people are very confused about the benefits/dangers of consuming soybeans and soy products, corn and corn products, and wheat and wheat products. I believe that when these staple foods are genetically modified, as so often is the case, they have the potential to be very harmful to human health. Over 80 percent of genetically engineered crops grown worldwide are modified to tolerate being sprayed with the extremely dangerous **glyphosate** herbicide. The Genetic Literacy Project cited ten scientific studies proving that GMOs can be harmful to human health. Here is what these studies found:

1. Multiple toxins from GMOs were detected in maternal and fetal blood.

2. DNA from genetically modified crops can be transferred to the humans who eat them.

3. Gluten disorders are linked to GMOs.

4. Tumors in rats are linked to genetically modified corn.

5. Glyphosate induces human breast cancer growth via estrogen receptors.

6. Glyphosate is linked to birth defects.

7. Glyphosate is linked to autism, Parkinson's and Alzheimer's.

8. Chronically ill patients have higher glyphosate levels than healthy humans.

9. GMO animal feed is linked to severe stomach inflammation and enlarged uteri in pigs.

10. Assessments that minimize GMO risk are based on very little scientific evidence, in the sense that the testing methods recommended are not adequate to ensure safety.

If you would like more information regarding the above studies please visit the website: www.genetic literacyproject.org.

When in doubt, it is always best to avoid potentially harmful carcinogenic foods. However, I believe it is relatively safe to consume organically grown soybeans, corn, and wheat, unless you have an allergy or sensitivity to these particular foods.

Soy has become particularly controversial with regard to its phytoestrogen nature (plant-derived estrogenic compounds). Many people believe soy-derived phytoestrogen to be a cancer-promoting substance. Whereas this may be true with regard to genetically modified soy, when we look to the cultures that have been consuming soy in the form of edamame (soybeans), tofu, and miso over many, many generations, such as the Japanese culture, we find that they currently have, and have had over many, many generations, a very low percentage of all types of cancer when compared with western societies. The low presence of cancer in the Japanese culture would indicate that soy is not the culprit. The real culprit is the way we are genetically modifying and processing soy in the West. Therefore, I believe that processed soy products such as soy hot dogs, other soy mock meats, soy cheeses, and other processed soy products should also be avoided.

EXCITOTOXINS

Excitotoxins, better known as neurotoxins, are food additives that are dangerous to brain function. These are addictive substances that literally excite neurons to death. Excitotoxins can be found in many different packaged foods in our grocery stores. The most notably recognized excitotoxins are monosodium glutamate and aspartame.

Monosodium glutamate

Monosodium glutamate (MSG) was isolated from kombu seaweed in 1908 by a Japanese biochemist. Shortly after its discovery, it was developed as the basis of a multi-million-dollar international industry. Following the Second World War, American food manufacturers became aware of this taste enhancing substance and began adding it to the foods they produced. At this time, they thought it was so safe that they began to add it to baby food. Neuroscientists presumed that glutamate provided the brain with energy. However, when two

ADDITIVES THAT CONTAIN MSG	ADDITIVES THAT OFTEN CONTAIN MSG
Monosodium glutamate	Malt extract
Hydrolyzed vegetable protein	Malt flavoring
Hydrolyzed protein	Bouillon
Hydrolyzed plant protein	Broth
Plant protein extract	Stock
Sodium caseinate	Flavoring
Calcium caseinate	Seasoning
Yeast extract	Spices
Textured protein	
Autolyzed yeast	
Hydrolyzed oat flour	

ophthalmologists, Newhouse and Lucas, decided to use MSG in a 1957 experiment to study an eye disease in mice, they were horrified to find that MSG had destroyed all the nerve cells in the inner eyes of the mice. Their findings related not only to nerve destruction in the eyes, but also to neuron damage in the brains of the young mice.

It is best to avoid consuming MSG, and all additives containing MSG, and limit or completely avoid additives that often contain MSG.

Aspartame

Aspartame is a methyl ester of aspartic acid/phenylalanine. Aspartame is the main ingredient of artificial sweeteners such as Nutra-Sweet and Equal, and is also one of the main ingredients found in chewing gum. Aspartame is the main sweetener used in many sugar-free/light foods, especially diet sodas. Like MSG, aspartame is another excitotoxin known to cause neuron damage, and is also an addictive substance that can alter brain chemistry. This substance should be avoided. Read your food labels!

BPA (BISPHENOL A)

✂ If you would like more information on excitotoxins, a good read is *Excitotoxins: The Taste That Kills*, by Russel L. Blaylock, MD.

Bisphenol A is a synthetic compound used in the production of plastic bottles and plastic storage containers, and in the lining of canned foods. This synthetic compound has been in commercial use since 1957, and the 2003–2004 National Health and Nutrition Examination Survey (NHANES III) conducted by the Centers for Disease Control and Prevention (CDC) found detectable levels of BPA in 93 percent of 2,517 urine samples from people six years and older. Other studies have shown that bisphenol A is a danger to human health. BPA has the tendency to break down, and leach into foods, and heating foods in plastic containers breaks down the chemical at a faster rate.

Bisphenol A is a danger to human health because when it enters the body, it mimics the hormone estrogen, making it a potential hormone disrupter and a danger to the endocrine system, and also a potentially cancer-causing substance. It is important to choose plastic containers and canned foods that clearly state they are BPA-free, and also try to choose glass or stainless-steel containers over plastic whenever possible.

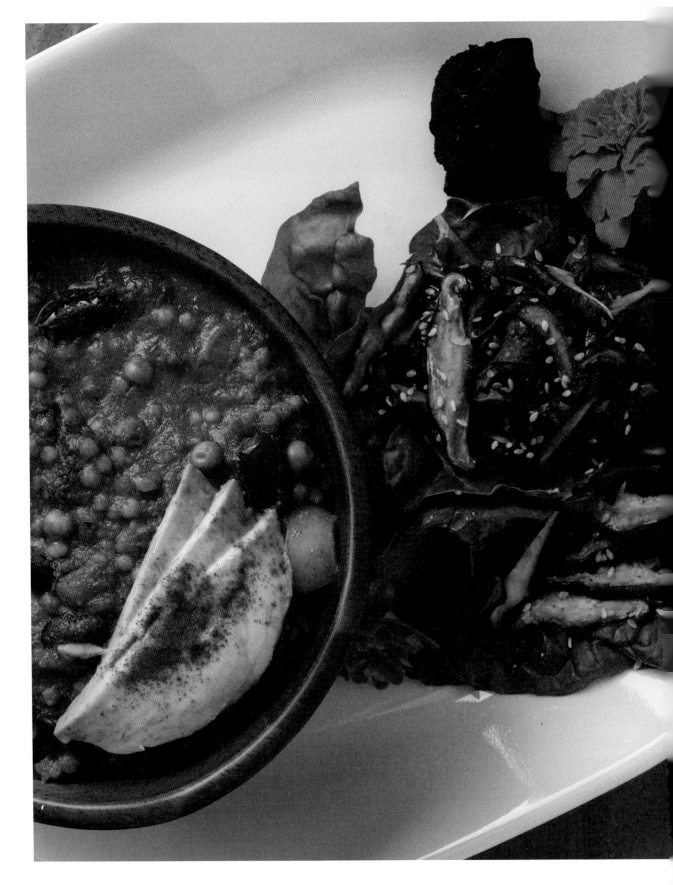

Preparing for a Whole Food, Plant-Based Lifestyle

READING FOOD LABELS

When reading food labels, the first thing to look at is the serving size, which is clearly indicated near the top of the label. Then compare the serving size from the label to the actual size of the serving of food that you intend to consume from the package. If the amount you intend to consume is the same as the serving size, you know that all the nutrient amounts you will be consuming are as listed on the label. The number of calories indicated will let you know how much energy is coming from that particular serving size.

Next look at the percent daily value (% Daily Value). This ranges on a scale from 0 to 100 percent; anything above 15 percent daily value (DV) shows that you are getting a lot of that particular nutrient, and anything below 5 percent DV is low in that particular nutrient. Look for percentages high in vitamins, minerals, and fiber, and percentages low in saturated fat, sodium, and sugar.

Let's take a look at the following food labels, the label on the left is the old nutrition fact label and the one on the right is the updated version. The improvements to the updated label make it easier to understand, and calories per serving size are easy to find. The new label clearly states how much added sugar this particular food contains. The following food label demonstrates that this food is high

Nutrition Facts

Serving Size 2/3 cup (55g)
Servings Per Container About 8

Amount Per Serving

Calories 230	Calories from Fat 72

	% Daily Value*
Total Fat 8g	**12%**
Saturated Fat 1g	**5%**
Trans Fat 0g	
Cholesterol 0mg	**0%**
Sodium 160mg	**7%**
Total Carbohydrate 37g	**12%**
Dietary Fiber 4g	**16%**
Sugars 1g	
Protein 3g	

Vitamin A	10%
Vitamin C	8%
Calcium	20%
Iron	45%

* Percent Daily Values are based on a 2,000 calorie diet. Your daily value may be higher or lower depending on your calorie needs.

	Calories:	2,000	2,500
Total Fat	Less than	65g	80g
Sat Fat	Less than	20g	25g
Cholesterol	Less than	300mg	300mg
Sodium	Less than	2,400mg	2,400mg
Total Carbohydrate		300g	375g
Dietary Fiber		25g	30g

Nutrition Facts

8 servings per container

Serving size	**2/3 cup (55g)**

Amount per serving

Calories	**230**

	% Daily Value*
Total Fat 8g	**10%**
Saturated Fat 1g	**5%**
Trans Fat 0g	
Cholesterol 0mg	**0%**
Sodium 160mg	**7%**
Total Carbohydrate 37g	**13%**
Dietary Fiber 4g	**14%**
Total Sugars 12g	
Includes 10g Added Sugars	**20%**
Protein 3g	

Vitamin D 2mcg	10%
Calcium 260mg	20%
Iron 8mg	45%
Potassium 235mg	6%

* The % Daily Value (DV) tells you how much a nutrient in a serving of food contributes to a daily diet. 2,000 calories a day is used for general nutrition advice.

These label examples are from the U.S. Food & Drug administration and can be found on the fda.gov website.

❀ *Tip:* When buying tinned/canned foods look for products that state "BPA-free." BPA (bisphenol A) is a very dangerous chemical that is used in the lining of tinned/canned foods, baby bottles, and other plastic containers. This chemical leaks into the foods we consume and is a potential hormone disrupter.

in important nutrients such as iron and calcium, and contains a moderate to high amount of carbohydrates and fiber. A large portion of the carbohydrates are from added sugars, making it very high in sugars, at 20 percent of the daily value.

WHAT TO ORDER WHEN EATING OUT

When I tell people that I do not eat animal products, and that I only consume whole plants foods, I always get the question, "What do you order when you eat out?" You may even be asking yourself the same question. Too many people succumb to the temptation of giving up what they believe in, to cheat or overindulge when socializing, only to regret it afterward. You do not have to forgo your social life to stick to a whole food, plant-based diet. Actually, sticking to a whole food, plant-based diet is really very simple. Regardless of the type of venue in which you choose to dine, you can always find vegan options on the menu. You can even call ahead or go online to preview the menu. Occasionally, the chef may even prepare something special for you if you ask nicely.

WHEN EATING OUT

Below are some options I choose when eating out:

Steak House

If there is a vegetable or bean soup on the menu, I will choose that along with a salad (no cheese please!). For my main course, I will choose from the side dishes, maybe a baked potato and fresh steamed or sautéed vegetables.

Italian Restaurant

Start with a vegetable or bean soup and salad, followed by a pasta with marinara sauce, again passing on the cheese. Also, look at the side dishes. At one particular restaurant, I ordered sides of white beans, sautéed broccolini, and marinara sauce, mixed them all together, and it was delicious.

Thai Restaurant

I like to order steamed brown rice and stir fry vegetables, of course you can add tofu if you like. Typically, you will also find great soups with rice noodles, and plenty of vegetables.

Japanese

Below I have listed many of the vegetable sushi rolls, usually found in Japanese restaurants. They are typically found on the menu as maki rolls. (Maki is a type of roll in which the seaweed wrap is on the outside of the roll).

Kappa (maki)	Kampyo (maki)
Avocado (maki)	Yuba (maki)
Shitake (maki)	Oshinko (maki)
Horenso (maki)	Ume (maki)

There are also many tofu dishes and side dishes to choose from. Check out www.vegi-etokyo.com.

French Restaurant

Dining at a French restaurant might include starting with a vegetable soup, followed by a salad and sides of fresh, streamed or sautéed vegetables and potatoes.

WHEN EATING OUT *(continued)*

German Restaurant

I would order steamed vegetables, potatoes, and lots of sauerkraut (which I love, and which is full of healthy probiotics).

Greek Restaurant

Soup, salad, hummus, olives, eggplant puree, fava-bean puree and extra vegetables for dipping.

Mexican Restaurant

Bean soup, and salad, bean burrito or tacos without cheese and sour cream. Also, there are always side-dish options such as rice, beans, mushrooms, guacamole, and salsas.

Indian Restaurant

I would choose a vegetable soup, salad, and yellow lentils with garlic, or chickpeas with garam masala, served with brown basmati or jasmine rice if available

Middle Eastern Restaurant

Plenty of choices here: lentil soup, baked falafel, hummus, fattoush salad, tabbouleh, baba ghanoush, and vegetable and rice stuffed grape leaves.

As you can see, eating a plant-based diet does not limit you to a certain type of restaurant. There are many healthy options to choose from wherever you go.

WHAT TO PREPARE FOR A ROAD TRIP

Road trips can be challenging and exhausting, especially if you are not fueling your body with the right foods. Rest stops and fast food establishments line the highways, so it is always best to start your journey off well stocked with healthy road-trip snacks to munch on along the way. First, make sure you have a large enough cooler in which to refrigerate your goodies. Water is always the best choice for hydration.

FOR THE ROAD

Here are some of the snacks I like to prepare ahead of time:

Small baked white potatoes

Small baked sweet potatoes

Small bowls of cooked quinoa or brown rice topped with chopped salad (mix of beets, carrots, celery, cucumber and onion) and lemon juice

Live raw bars

Live power bars

Ziploc bags full of sliced veggies, such as carrots, cucumbers, celery, and bell peppers

Container of hummus for dipping your sliced veggies

Sprouted sunflower seeds

Sprouted pumpkin seeds

Banana energy balls (see recipe on page 257)

Cumin curry crackers (see recipe on page 262)

Muffins (see recipes on pages 136, 137, 140, 144)

Plant Power Protein-Rich Granola (see recipe on page 130)

Hemp bites

Chia bites

Fresh fruit: apples, bananas, peaches, pears, nectarines, tangerines

Boxed cereal, something low in sugar and high in fiber, such as Engine 2, Rip's Big Bowl banana walnut cereal, Kashi, or muesli. Just make sure what you choose is 5 grams of sugar or less per ½-cup serving

Boxed/cartoned milk, unsweetened hemp or almond. You can make your own, but it won't last as long on the road

❋ Also, you will need utensils, paper bowls, and napkins. It is always a good idea to take along baby wipes too!

Tip: Always keep BPA-free tinned/canned or cartoned varieties available to prepare quick and easy meals.

WHAT TO STOCK IN YOUR PANTRY

The following is a list of everything you will need to stock your pantry for a whole food, plant-based lifestyle. By keeping healthy supplies close at hand, you will always be well prepared to make delicious plant-based meals.

WHAT TO STOCK *in Your Pantry*

WHOLE GRAINS

Gluten Free

Amaranth	Kasha	Wild rice	Kamut
Brown basmati rice	Millet	Whole rolled oats	Rye berries
Brown jasmine rice	Quinoa	*Contains Gluten*	Rye flakes
Brown rice, long grain	Red rice	Barley flakes	Spelt berries
Brown rice, short grain	Sorghum	Brown barley	Wheat berries
Buckwheat	Sprouted brown rice	Bulgur	Wheat flakes
	Steel-cut oats	Farro	Whole-wheat
	Teff		couscous

BEANS AND LENTILS

Adzuki beans	Butter/lima beans	Green lentils	Pinto beans
Cannellini beans	Dahl	Green split peas	Red beans
Black beans	Dry pigeon peas	Fava beans	Red lentils
Black-eyed peas	Garbanzo beans	Kidney beans	Sprouted lentils
Black lentils	(chickpeas)	Mung beans	Yellow split peas
	Great northern beans		

FRESH HERBS

Basil	Dill	Oregano	Sage
Chives	Mint	Parsley	Tarragon
Cilantro	Marjoram	Rosemary	Thyme

WHAT TO STOCK *in Your Pantry* (continued)

SPICES

Allspice	Cloves	Marjoram	Seaweed gomasio
Basil	Coriander	Nutmeg	Smoked paprika
Bay leaves	Cumin	Onion powder	Smokey turmeric
Black pepper corns	Garlic powder	Oregano	Thyme
Cardamom	Ginger	Parsley	Turmeric
Cayenne	Garam Masala	Rosemary	Vanilla extract
Chili powder	Himalayan pink	Sage	
Cinnamon	sea salt	Saffron	

SUGARS AND SWEETENERS

Agave nectar	Coconut nectar	Coconut palm sugar

SUPER NUTS AND SEEDS *(always raw, preferably unsalted)*

Almonds	Hemp seeds	Pumpkin seeds	Sprouted sunflower
Brazil nuts	Flaxseeds	Sesame seeds	seeds
Cashews	Macadamia nuts	Sprouted pumpkin	Sunflower seeds
Chia seeds	Pecans	seeds	Walnuts
Hazelnuts	Pistachios		

SUPER NUT AND SEED BUTTERS

Organic peanut butter	Raw pumpkin	Raw sprouted	Sesame seed tahini
Raw almond butter	seed butter	pumpkin seed	Organic peanut butter
Raw cashew butter		butter	

OILS AND BUTTERS

Cacao butter	Hemp	Pumpkin seed
Coconut	Olive	Sesame

VINEGARS

Apple cider	Balsamic	Brown rice

WHAT TO STOCK *in Your Pantry* (continued)

CONDIMENTS AND MISCELLANEOUS

Baking powder
Baking soda
Bragg liquid amino acids
Chopped, roasted garlic

Chopped, roasted tomatoes
Coconut liquid amino acids
Gluten-free egg replacer
Ketchup

Low-sodium tamari sauce
Light coconut milk
Organic tempeh
Organic tofu
Sun-dried tomatoes

Roasted red bell peppers
Tomato paste
Vegan Worcestershire sauce
Vegetable stock
Whole-grain Dijon mustard

DRIED SUPER FRUIT

Apricots
Figs

Medjool dates
Raisins

Goji berries
Mulberries

Golden berries

DRIED SUPERFOODS AND POWDERS

Açaí berry powder
Cacao nibs
Camu camu powder

Chlorella powder
Maca powder
Matcha green tea powder

Moringa
Plant protein powder e.g. Hemp powder
Raw cacao powder

Spirulina powder
Vanilla bean extract powder

FLOURS

Buckwheat flour
Coconut flour
Garbanzo flour

Gluten-free all-purpose flour

Gluten-free oat flour
Millet flour

Sorghum flour
Quinoa flour

WHAT TO STOCK *in Your Freezer*

FROZEN FRUITS

Blueberries
Raspberries
Blackberries

Strawberries
Cranberries
Mango

Peaches
Pineapple
Bananas

Black cherries
Papaya

WHAT TO STOCK *in Your Refrigerator*

FROZEN VEGETABLES

Broccoli
Carrots

Green peas
Lima beans

Organic edamame
(soybeans)

Organic corn

FRESH VEGETABLES

The Most Nutritious Salad Greens

Arugula
Basil
Kale
Mint
Parsley
Romaine
Spinach
Swiss chard
Watercress

Vegetables to Top Your Salad

Avocado
Beets
Bell peppers
Carrots
Celery
Cucumber
Fennel
Green onions
(scallions)
Mushrooms
Onions
Radish

Red onions
Snap peas
Sprouted greens
Sweet onions
Tomatoes

Vegetables for Side Dishes

Asparagus
Bok choy
Broccoli
Butternut squash
Carrots
Cauliflower

Eggplant
Green beans
Fingerling potatoes
Kale
Mushrooms
Spinach
Sweet potatoes
Swiss chard
Red Potatoes
Russet potatoes
Yams
Yellow squash
Zucchini

FRESH FRUITS

Apples
Bananas
Blackberries
Black grapes
Blueberries
Cantaloupe

Cherries
Cranberries
Dragon fruit
Honeydew melon
Lemons
Limes

Mango
Nectarines
Oranges
Papaya
Passion fruit
Peaches

Pears
Pomegranates
Strawberries
Raspberries
Watermelon

Tip: Buy all the colors and varieties you can find. Always try to choose organic varieties first, local if possible, and try to purchase produce in season.

Cooking Your *Gluten-Free Grains*

Whole rolled oats	Also known as old fashioned oats, great in breads, cookies, and muffins	1 cup oats to 2 cups liquid	Bring to a slight boil and simmer for 5 to 10 minutes
Steel-cut oats	Creamy, chewy breakfast cereal	1 cup steel-cut oats to 3 cups liquid	Bring to a slight boil and simmer for 10 minutes
Kasha	Whole-roasted buckwheat groats, great in stuffing	1 cup kasha to 2 cups liquid	Bring to slight boil and simmer for 15–20 minutes
Buckwheat	My favorite breakfast cereal, creamy and delicious	1 cup buckwheat to 3 cups liquid	Bring to a slight boil and simmer for 10 minutes
Sorghum	A larger grain with a chewy texture, great in curries, soups, and salads	1 cup sorghum to 3 cups liquid	Bring to a slight boil, cover and simmer for 50–60 minutes
Teff	Great as a breakfast cereal, creamy and high in calcium	1 cup teff to 3 cups liquid	Bring water to a boil, add teff, and simmer for 15–20 minutes
Wild rice	Chewy but flavorful, great addition to soups	1 cup rice to 3 cups water	Rinse well before cooking, bring to a boil, simmer for 45 minutes
Quinoa	An ancient grain, versatile and high in protein	1 cup quinoa to 2 cups water	Rinse well before cooking, bring to a slight boil, simmer for 15–20 minutes
Millet	Easily digestible, similar to quinoa	1 cup millet to 2½ cups water	Simmer for 30 minutes, fluff, and let sit for 15 minutes
Amaranth	Sticky when cooked, I enjoy it as a cereal for breakfast	1 cup amaranth to 3 cups water	Bring to a boil and simmer for 25 minutes
Brown rice, long grain	Fluffs up when cooked	1 cup rice to 2 cups water	Rinse well before cooking, bring to a boil and cover, simmer for 45 minutes
Brown rice, short grain	Great for stir-frys and stuffing vegetables	1 cup rice to 2 cups water	Rinse well before cooking, bring to a boil and cover, simmer for 45 minutes
Brown jasmine rice	Aromatic fragrance, great with curries	1 cup rice to 2 cups water	Rinse well before cooking, simmer for 45 minutes
Brown basmati rice	Aromatic and flavorful	1 cup rice to 2 cups water	Please add bring to a boil, cover, and simmer for 45 minutes. Can be soaked for 20–30 minutes before cooking to soften the grain
Red rice	Nutty flavor, the most nutrient dense rice	1 cup rice to 2 cups water	Rinse well before cooking, bring to a boil and cover, simmer for 40 minutes

Cooking Your *Grains*

Farro	Great source of fiber with a nutty flavor	1 cup farro to 3 cups liquid	Bring to a boil and simmer covered for 10 minutes
Spelt berries	Easily digested ancient grain	1 cup spelt berries to 4 cups liquid	Soak overnight, drain, add water, bring to a boil, and simmer for 55 minutes
Barley flakes	Cooks similar to whole oats, great breakfast cereal	1 cup barley to 2 cups liquid	Bring to a slight boil and simmer for 10 minutes
Brown barley	Chewy, mild flavor, great in soups and added to stuffing for vegetables	1 cup barley to 3½ cups liquid	Bring to a slight boil and simmer for 25 minutes
Whole-wheat couscous	A nutty flavor, more nutritious than regular couscous because the outer bran layer is retained	1 cup couscous to 1½ cups liquid	Place couscous in a bowl and cover with boiled water and a pinch of salt, cover and let sit for 10 minutes.
Kamut	Chewy, buttery flavor	1 cup kamut to 3 cups liquid	Soak overnight, drain, add water, bring to a slight boil, and simmer for 45–50 minutes
Rye berries	Nutty flavor and texture, great in baked goods and stuffing	1 cup berries to 4 cups liquid	Soak overnight, bring to a slight boil, and simmer for 55 minutes
Wheat berries	High in protein and great in salads and stuffing	1 cup berries to 4 cups liquid	Soak overnight, drain, add water, bring to a boil, and simmer for 55 minutes
Wheat flakes	Rolled from wheat berries, great mixed with other cereal grains	1 cup flakes to 3 cups liquid	Bring to a slight boil and simmer for 25 minutes
Rye flakes	Rolled rye berries, great in baked goods or as a breakfast cereal	1 cup rye flakes to 3 cups liquid	Bring to a slight boil and simmer for 35 minutes
Bulgur	Partially cooked, cracked wheat used in tabbouleh	1 cup bulgur to 2½ cups liquid	Bring to a slight boil and simmer for 55 minutes

Cooking Your *Beans and Lentils*

Garbanzo beans	Irregular round shape with a creamy, nutty taste, great in hummus and veggie burgers	Soak overnight before cooking, 1 cup of beans to 3½ cups water	Simmer gently for 1½ hours, add salt ¾ of the way through cooking
Kidney beans	Red and shaped like a kidney with a meaty-like mild flavor, great in chili	Soak overnight before cooking, 1 cup of beans to 3½ cups water	Simmer gently for 1–1½ hours, add salt ¾ of the way through cooking
Pinto beans	Cream colored with streaks of brown, color changes when cooked; very creamy texture, great for bean dips	Soak overnight before cooking, 1 cup of beans to 3 ⅓ cups water	Simmer gently for 2 hours, add salt ¾ of the way through cooking.
Cannellini beans	Also known as white kidney beans, great for salads and Italian dishes	Soak overnight before cooking, 1 cup of beans to 3½ cups water	Simmer gently for 1½ hours, add salt ¾ of the way through cooking
Lima beans	Also called butter beans, mild, slightly sweet taste and a creamy texture, great in soups and casseroles	Soak overnight before cooking, 1 cup of beans to 3½ cups water	Simmer gently for 1 hour, add salt ¾ of the way through cooking
Adzuki beans	Also known as aduki beans, relatively easy to digest, a small reddish, brown bean with a nutty-like flavor	Soak overnight before cooking, 1 cup of beans to 3½ cups water	Simmer gently for 45–60 minutes, add salt ¾ of the way through cooking
Black beans	Very small black beans, great with cumin and garlic, salsas, guacamole, and in burgers, meaty and earthy	Soak overnight before cooking, 1 cup of beans to 3½ cups water	Simmer gently for 1½ hours, add salt ¾ of the way through cooking
Fava beans	Great mixed with oil, lemon, garlic, and cumin as a side dish to soups and salads, meaty texture	Soak overnight before cooking, 1 cup of beans to 3½ cups water	Simmer gently for 1½ hours, add salt ¾ of the way through cooking
Mung beans	Very easily digested, a small round green bean, great on salads and added to soups	No soaking required, 1 cup beans to 3 cups water	Simmer gently for 1¼ hours, add salt ¾ of the way through cooking
Red beans	Small, dark red bean, slightly sweet in flavor, try red beans and rice	Soak overnight before cooking, 1 cup beans to 3½ cups water	Simmer gently for 1½–2 hours, add salt ¾ of the way through cooking
Great northern beans	White beans, great for soups and hummus, with a mild, creamy, nutty flavor.	Soak overnight before cooking, 1 cup beans to 3½ cups liquid	Simmer gently for 1 hour, add salt ¾ of the way through cooking

Cooking Your **Beans and Lentils** (continued)

Black lentils	Black in color, great in salads and burgers	1 cup lentils to 1½ cups liquid	Bring to a boil, partially cover and simmer gently for 25–30 minutes, add salt ¾ of the way through cooking
Red lentils	Light pink in color and golden when cooked, great in curries and soups	1 cup lentils to 1½ cups liquid	Bring to a boil, partially cover, and simmer gently for 25 minutes, add salt ¾ of the way through cooking
Green lentils	Also known as brown lentils, add turmeric, cumin, and ginger and puree to make Indian dahl	1 cup lentils to 1½ cups liquid	Bring to a boil, partially cover, and simmer gently for 45–60 minutes, add salt ¾ of the way through cooking
Yellow split peas	Soft and mild tasting, great in curried dishes and soups, with lemon and cumin	1 cup peas to 1½ cups liquid	Bring to a boil, partially cover, and simmer gently for 45–60 minutes, add salt ¾ of the way through cooking
Green split peas	Everyone loves split-pea soup!	1 cup peas to 1½ cups liquid	Bring to a boil, partially cover, and simmer gently for 45–60 minutes, add salt ¾ of the way through cooking
Black-eyed peas	Small beige beans with distinctive black marks	1 cup peas to 1½ cups liquid	Bring to a boil, partially cover, and simmer gently for 1 hour, add salt ¾ of the way through cooking
Dahl	An Indian legume with a mild flavor, great mixed with spices, onions, and tomatoes	1 cup dahl to 1½ cups liquid	Bring to a boil, reduce to a simmer, partially cover, and cook for 30–40 minutes
Dry pigeon peas	Light brown in color, a staple of the Caribbean	1 cup dry pigeon peas to 2½ cups liquid	Bring to a boil, reduce to simmer, cover and cook for 1½ hours, until tender

Tip: To add flavor to your beans, add garlic and a bay leaf at the beginning of cooking. To add flavor to your lentils, cook them in vegetable broth with a bay leaf, a little minced garlic, and chopped onion.

KITCHEN APPLIANCES REQUIRED

Live Simply Plant-Based requires no more than a few appliances:

- Good blender ~ Vitamix is the best, but a NutriBullet pro also works well. Used for blending smoothies, drinks, juices and dressings.
- Juicer ~ Breville juicers work well.
- Food processor ~ For making burgers, pizza base, crackers, dips, sauces, puddings, creams, nut cheeses, and spreads.
- Food Mixer ~ Great for making Live Bars and burgers.

You can mix by hand, but using a mixer is quicker and easier.

- Coffee grinder ~ For grinding seeds, herbs, and making flours.
- Whisk ~ For making chia puddings. A hand whisk will do.
- Chopper ~ For chopping vegetables. Best invention ever!

Other items required

- Measuring cups
- Measuring spoons
- Vegetable peeler
- Lemon/lime juicer/squeezer

- Orange juicer/squeezer
- Jars and glass storage containers
- Citrus zester or fine grater

RICE

The benefits of brown rice versus white rice are well known. In case you are not sure of the benefits, here are a few facts. White rice is a processed grain, and works as a simple carbohydrate. White rice is low in nutrient value and spikes blood sugar, causing the pancreas to work harder. Brown rice, on the other hand, has been minimally processed, is high in fiber, rich in vitamins and minerals, and helps to balance blood sugar levels, so the pancreas does not have to work so hard.

There is a lot of confusing information regarding arsenic levels in rice. Please refer to the following information regarding brands and sources that have been tested and shown to contain the least amount of arsenic.

Lundberg Farms rice has been shown to contain lower amounts of arsenic than many other brands. Aromatic rices, such as brown basmati, brown jasmine, red rice, and black rice, have lower arsenic levels than most others. Rice from California, India, and Pakistan has lower levels of arsenic compared to rice produced in the southern regions of the U.S. This is because, thirty years ago, tons of arsenic were spread on cotton fields in the southern states where rice is now grown. If you are wondering which color rice is the most nutrient-dense—brown, red, or black—the answer is red rice. It contains up to ten times more antioxidants than brown rice.

SUPERFOODS

Superfood is a widely used term to describe extremely nutrient-dense foods. I believe that all whole plant foods are superfoods, but here are some of my favorites:

Tip: I like to soak my rice in vegetable stock and/or water the night before cooking to neutralize any phytic acid, and then cook it in the same liquid the next day. See **Stocking Your Pantry** for correct information on amounts of liquid to rice. Generally, it will be 1 cup rice to 2 cups liquid.

Tip: To make rice milk, follow my nut and seed milk instructions and substitute 1 cup cooked brown rice for 1 cup nuts or seeds.

Tip: To add flavor to rice, millet, sorghum, or quinoa, cook it in vegetable stock. To add extra flavor to rice, add garlic, ginger, shiitake mushrooms, and a bay leaf at the beginning of cooking.

Amaranth

Tip: If you would like to cook amaranth, millet, or teff to be fluffy like quinoa, heat a large skillet over medium heat, and toast grain for a few minutes first before cooking. Try not to let it burn. Amaranth will turn golden, and millet will turn tan.

Amaranth looks like a grain, and tastes nutty and grainy, but is not really a grain. It is actually the seed of a tall, weed-like flower. Today amaranth is known as an ancient grain, due to its history as a staple food of the Aztecs, dating back eight thousand years. Amaranth is naturally gluten-free, and its proteins are easily digested. It can be ground into flour and used in baking, heated on the stove top with water or plant milk and made into a delicious porridge, or toasted and cooked into a fluffy, quinoa-like texture.

Amaranth is a great source of protein and fiber, providing 9 grams of protein per cup, cooked. Amaranth is rich in calcium, magnesium, manganese, potassium, iron, phosphorus, and B6. It is also a good source of riboflavin (B2), folate, thiamin (B1), and vitamin C. For those who have sensitive digestive systems when consuming grains, soaking them before cooking, preferably overnight, makes them easier to digest, by releasing digestive inhibitors such as phytic acid. If you prefer to sprout your grains, this will take longer, but you will reap even more nutritional benefits. Amaranth is an anti-inflammatory, bone-building, cholesterol-lowering and a blood sugar-stabilizing superfood.

Chia Seeds

Chia seeds, are an ancient staple of the Aztecs and the Mayans, and a superfood in their own right. They have a nutty flavor and are super-dense in nutrients. A relative of the mint family of plants, they are found predominantly in southern Mexico. Chia seeds are abundant in omega-3 fatty acids, even more so than flaxseeds, and do not need to be ground down to reap the benefit of these important nutrients.

Chia seeds have a long shelf life, and do need to be refrigerated once opened. When mixed with water or plant milk, chia forms a gel-like, pudding consistency. Chia can also be sprinkled on cereals, and salads. The seeds slow down the rate at which the body breaks down carbohydrates into sugar, therefore providing long, sustained energy. One ounce of chia seeds provides 5 grams of protein and almost 7 grams of fiber. Besides being rich in calcium, magnesium, and iron, chia seeds provide a good source of phosphorus, manganese, copper, molybdenum, niacin, and zinc. Check out my chia pudding recipes!

Buckwheat

Despite its name, buckwheat does not contain any wheat and is, therefore, gluten-free. It is an ancient grain, contains lower levels of phytic acid than most other grains, and is very easily digested. With an intense flavor, similar to hops, buckwheat is not really a grain, but actually the seed of a type of fruit. Its uses are many: it can be made into a tasty porridge, it is delicious in pancakes, and it can be ground into a flour for use in baking. In addition to being a rich source of phosphorus, potassium, magnesium, iron, and B6, it is high in dietary fiber and a good source of protein. Buckwheat helps lower cholesterol levels, lowers blood pressure, contains antioxidants, and contains easily digestible proteins. Buckwheat does not need to be soaked before cooking, but can be, and requires less soaking time than other grains. See my high energy breakfast recipes!

Hemp Seeds

Hemp seeds do not require soaking before consuming. They are an excellent source of easily digestible protein, and have a delicious nutty-like flavor. They are a great way of adding protein to smoothies, and cereals, and can easily be made into a plant milk with a creamy texture. Hemp seeds are made up of 33 percent protein, and are rich in essential fatty acids. They also contain all eight essential amino acids, making them a complete protein. Besides being a great source of fiber, and rich in phosphorus, magnesium, zinc, vitamin E, and iron, they also contain many other nutrients. Hemp seeds help increase immunity and relieve constipation. Unlike animal protein, hemp seeds are anti-inflammatory in nature, heart strengthening, and cancer fighting, which is why hemp seeds are a superfood!

Walnuts

Walnuts are the seeds of the genus Juglans (walnut tree) family, and are considered a food for the brain due to their uncanny appearance, resembling the human brain. They contain omega-3 fatty acids, which are known to assist in neurotransmission within the brain. They have a bitter, rich flavor, and are delicious topped on cereals and salads, used in baking, or roasted or toasted. Walnuts are a rich source of calcium, magnesium, phosphorus, potassium, manganese, zinc, copper, and selenium. They also contain B vitamins, and vitamins A, E, C, and K. You can soak them, and make a creamy, delicious walnut milk. Walnuts are not only brain food, but are also heart healthy, anti-inflammatory, bone-building, and help stabilize blood sugar. Walnuts are a metabolism booster, and have cancer preventing properties. Eat your walnuts!

Pumpkin Seeds

Pumpkin seeds date all the way back to the Aztecs of central Mexico. They are amazing little powerhouses, packed with many nutritional benefits. Pumpkin seeds are a good source of protein, making up 30 percent of their nutritional content, with 28 grams in every cup. Rich in magnesium, manganese, phosphorus, tryptophan, copper, iron, and zinc, pumpkin seeds also contain B vitamins and vitamin A. Pumpkin seeds have a relaxing effect on the body, helping to induce a good night's sleep. They help lower cholesterol levels, are bone building, and help to lower blood pressure. Pumpkin seeds are also known to prevent prostate cancer, kidney stones, and speed up metabolism. You can presoak them, roast/toast them, make them into pumpkin seed butter, and use them to top cereals and salads. You can also sprout them or purchase them already sprouted. Don't miss out on this amazing superfood!

Spirulina

Spirulina is known as nature's superfood. It is a type of blue-green algae found growing on the coast of Kona, Hawaii, in fresh aquifers, as well as other regions in the world. Spirulina has a fishy smell and a bitter strong flavor, but packs a massive punch when it comes to nutrient content. Made up of 60 percent protein, it is loaded with beta carotene, vitamins K1, K2, B12 (an important nutrient for vegans), and iron. Spirulina is a good source of magnesium, manganese, and sodium. It is higher in beta carotene than carrots, and contains substantially more iron than spinach. Rich in antioxidants, spirulina is a great source of chlorophyll a, gamma linolenic acid (GLA), zeaxanthin, and phycocyanin. Spirulina helps the body eliminate heavy metals and toxins, increases immunity, regulates blood pressure, and lowers cholesterol. It also is anti-inflammatory, alkaline, protects the liver, eliminates candida, helps increase focus, preserves bone health, and boosts metabolism. Spirulina can be added to smoothies and juices, as well as nutrition bars, and baked goods. See my liquid nutrition recipes!

Tip: Be aware that some studies have shown that certain varieties of spirulina grown in China contain toxic contaminants.

Chlorella

Chlorella is an ancient species of algae indigenous to the Far East. Like spirulina, it is a fresh-water, blue-green algae. Its odor is not as pungent as spirulina, and its taste is a little milder. Chlorella is a powerhouse of nutrients, and is loaded with chlorophyll. It is super-rich in vitamin A, B vitamins, and vitamin C. It is also rich in magnesium, sodium, iron, and zinc. Chlorella is also a great protein source, containing 16 grams per ounce, and is rich in essential and non-essential amino acids. In addition to assisting in detoxing the body by binding to harmful toxins and eliminating them from the body, Chlorella also boosts the immune system, speeds up metabolism, and has cancer-fighting properties. Chlorella complements spirulina, so you can combine them for a super nutrient boost. Chlorella can be added to smoothies and juices, to breakfast grains, and teas. Eat and drink your greens!

Maca Root

Maca helps to regulate hormone levels, increases libido, helps ease menopause symptoms . . .

The botanical name for maca root is Lepidium meyenii, and it grows at very high altitude in the Andes of central Peru. Maca root has a pleasant, sweet nutty-like flavor resembling its scent. Although the maca plant resembles a cruciferous vegetable, the root of the plant is the most edible part, and is usually dried and ground into a powder. Maca root is extremely nutrient dense: rich in vitamin C, copper, iron, potassium, vitamin B6, and manganese, it is also a good source of protein and carbohydrates, and contains polyphenols and glucosinolates. Maca helps to regulate hormone levels, increases libido, helps ease menopause symptoms, reduces anxiety and depression, and improves well-being. Maca root is also energy-boosting, and may be beneficial to prostate health. The powder can be added to juices and smoothies, topped on breakfast cereals, used in nutrition bars, and baked in foods. Although maca root is probably safe for most people, it is a goitrogen, which can lower thyroid function, so people with hypothyroidism should probably limit or avoid using maca root.

Matcha Green Tea

Matcha green tea powder is the best quality green tea powder available. Today matcha green tea leaves are grown predominantly in Japan, but date back to the Tang Dynasty of China. In the 1100s, matcha green tea plants were taken to Japan, where one of the richest sources of matcha green tea grows today. The leaves are harvested and finely ground into a beautiful, green, fragrant powder. Matcha green tea powder contains over one hundred times more antioxidants than regular green tea. It is rich in chlorophyll, vitamin C, magnesium, selenium, chromium, and zinc. It boosts the metabolism, allowing you to burn more calories at a faster rate. Matcha green tea powder increases energy, but also has a calming effect on the mind and body. It is detoxifying, increases immunity, lowers cholesterol, and regulates blood glucose. Add it to smoothies and juices, puddings, baked goods, nutrition bars, or enjoy simply as a tea. Matcha health!

Sweet Potato

The simple sweet potato; who knew it had so many nutritional benefits! A sweet potato is not a yam, as many people may think. A yam is higher in starch and calories, with lower antioxidant content. Sweet potatoes are packed full of vitamin A, and no other food compares to its vitamin A level. Sweet potatoes also rank low on the glycemic index, making them a great choice for those who have problems stabilizing their blood sugar. Sweet potatoes are rich in potassium, manganese, vitamin C, and B6, and are high in fiber, and anti-inflammatory in nature. They are also beneficial in keeping the skin healthy, due to their high retinol content. Sweet potatoes have cancer fighting properties, lower cholesterol levels, and help support a healthy prostate. Eat them raw, bake them, roast them, make them into soups, pies, or veggie burgers. See my recipes!

Sweet potatoes have cancer fighting properties, lower cholesterol levels, and help support a healthy prostate.

Lemons and Limes

Beautifully bright yellow and green, fragrant and flavorful little powerhouses of nutrition, lemons and limes are super-high in vitamin C, citric acid, polyphenols and phytochemicals, potassium, and fiber. Lemons are higher in sugar than limes, making them a little sweeter to the taste. They both share the same health benefits, boosting the immune system, increasing digestion, and speeding up the recovery from injury and surgery. They also help increase circulation, and have cancer fighting properties. Lemons are slightly more nutrient dense, but I consider both to be super-foods. They have so many culinary uses, and the zest from the peel of these incredible fruits also contains beneficial nutrients. Check out my liquid nutrition recipes for a vitamin C boost!

Aloe Vera

Aloe vera comes from the Asphodelaceae family, and is indigenous to dry regions of the world. The botanical name for aloe vera is Aloe barbadensis Miller. The plant dates back thousands of years, and is well known for its medicinal properties. The plant is green in color, its leaves are long and triangular in shape with thorn-like edges. Aloe vera contains seven of the eight essential amino acids, and twenty of the twenty-two non-essential amino acids, because it contains salicylic acid, as well as fatty acids, aloe vera possesses anti-bacterial, anti-inflammatory, and analgesic properties.

It has two hormones that assist in wound healing, and contains eight different enzymes which aid in the breakdown of sugars and fats. It also provides the minerals calcium, magnesium, manganese, potassium, selenium, sodium, copper, and zinc. This amazing plant also contains B12 (a very important nutrient to a plant-based diet), choline, folic acid, and vitamins A, C, and E. So, you can understand why I have incorporated this whole food into my lifestyle.

You will find a chunk of fresh aloe **inner fillet** regularly added to my smoothie/juice recipes. Wash the outer leaf well and slice off an inch-long chunk. Then slice off the thorny sides, carefully remove one side of the outer leaf, then the other, rinse off some of the sap-like substance (this ensures that you are not ingesting too much aloin, a bitter yellow compound known to have a laxative effect), and drop it into your Vitamix or NutriBullet along with your other whole-plant ingredients.

Avocado

The avocado is indigenous to Central America, and was discovered in the 16th century. Today avocado is grown in many regions of the world, and is well known for its nutritional benefits. The avocado is an amazing superfood! It has a smooth, creamy texture and flavor and, although considered a fruit, is extremely low in sugar. The avocado is rich in healthy monounsaturated fats and high in dietary fiber, potassium, phosphorus, magnesium, vitamin C, B vitamins, vitamin A, vitamin K, and iron. Avocado is also a good source of polyun-saturated fat, zinc, copper, manganese, and vitamin E. Avocado is anti-inflammatory, helps to keep joints healthy, protects the heart, lowers cholesterol, stabilizes blood sugar, and boosts metabolism.

Use avocado to make guacamole. It is also delicious as a salad or breakfast accompaniment, and adds a creamy thickness to smoothies, dressings, and toppings. Enjoy the many benefits of this delicious superfood!

Watercress

According to a study published by the Centers for Disease Control and Prevention, watercress is considered a superfood powerhouse due to its nutrient density, and I agree. Watercress is an aquatic plant species grown near slow-moving streams and springs, and is native to Asia and Europe. It has a rich, dark green color with flat round leaves, and a slightly spicy, peppery flavor. Watercress is a rich source of vitamin K, vitamin C, vitamin A, calcium, and omega-3 and omega-6 fatty acids. It also contains protein, B vitamins, phosphorus, potassium, manganese, and copper. Watercress may help lower blood pressure, strengthens bones and teeth, helps to prevent

Watercress may help lower blood pressure, strengthens bones and teeth, helps to prevent osteoporosis . . .

osteoporosis, keeps skin, hair, and nails healthy, has anti-inflammatory benefits, and may reduce the risk of colon-related diseases. Try one of my watercress salads!

Blueberries

Blueberries are native to North America, and date back to pre-colonial times. They are a rich blue-purple color when ripened, and deliciously sweet to the taste. Blueberries contain one of the highest amounts of antioxidants of any fruit or vegetable. Rich in vitamin C, vitamin K, and manganese, they are also high in dietary fiber, and low in calories. Blueberries are also a good source of calcium, magnesium, zinc, iron, and B6. Their vitamin C content assists in maintaining healthy collagen, preventing the skin from losing elasticity. Their minerals and vitamin K levels help to keep bones healthy. Blueberries also have heart-protective properties, and may protect against free-radical damage. Blueberries aid digestion, are colon protective, and help balance blood glucose. Use them as a topping on whole grains or salads, add them to breads, muffins, and pancakes, or enjoy them solo!

Bananas

One average-size banana equals close to 110 calories and almost 30 grams of carbohydrates. So bananas are an excellent source of quick energy, the perfect food to grab on the go, making them probably the most popular fruit consumed in the United States and around the world. Even though bananas are grown in tropical regions like Africa, Latin America, and the Caribbean, they actually originated in Southeast Asia and Oceania, and were introduced to America by Portuguese sailors. Bananas are a super-rich source of potassium, and are high in sugar, making them a good pre, or post workout snack. Bananas are a great source of vitamin C, B6, magnesium, dietary fiber, folate, manganese, choline and phytosterols.

Bananas are heart healthy, anti-inflammatory, strengthening to the nervous system, and beneficial to the digestive system. Eat your bananas!

Red Cabbage

The Latin name for cabbage, *bassica*, originated from the Celtic word, *bresic*, indicating that cabbage dates back to Celtic times, and may have been introduced to the Mediterranean by the Celts during an invasion. Red cabbage contains double the amount of iron found in green cabbage, and ten times more vitamin A. Red cabbage is extremely low in calories and very high in vitamin C, making it anti-inflammatory and collagen building. Red cabbage is also rich in vitamin A and protective to eye health. It is also a good source of vitamin K, assisting with blood clotting and helping build strong bones. The red pigment of the cabbage contains flavonoids and cyanidin, and these compounds work as antioxidants that may help prevent some types of cancers. Red cabbage is also a great source of dietary fiber, helping protect against colon-related disease.

Red cabbage contains double the amount of iron found in green cabbage, and ten times more vitamin A.

Shiitake Mushrooms

The shiitake mushroom has a long history as a medicinal food. It dates back over 100 million years to the mountains of Japan, Taiwan, Indonesia, and China. Shiitake mushrooms are a nutrient-rich source of B vitamins, and vitamins C and D, along with the minerals potassium, magnesium, phosphorus, manganese, iron, and zinc. They are also a good source of dietary fiber, and contain health protecting antioxidants. These powerful mushrooms are beneficial to weight loss, and are bone strengthening and anti-inflammatory in nature. Shiitake mushrooms have cancer-fighting properties, and help improve circulation and digestion. Their rich B-vitamin content makes them a great source of energy, and just a small amount can add a powerful punch to your health. Try chopping them and adding them to your rice when cooking; delicious in soups, and burgers, they add flavor as well as nutrition!

Onions

Food historians believe that onions originated in central Asia and are one of the oldest-known vegetables, dating back five thousand years, long before farming was invented. Onions were easily transported and non-perishable, and could be dried for later use to prevent dehydration. Onions were also a great nutrition source when other food was scarce. Knowledge of their medicinal properties dates back to over two thousand years ago in India, where they were used as a diuretic and to strengthen the heart, digestive system, eyes, and joints. Onions are nutrient rich in Vitamin C, flavonoids, and phytochemicals, and they also contain sulphur compounds believed to have cancer-fighting properties. Vitamin C makes onions a great immunity booster. The flavonoid quercetin is a powerful antioxidant with anti-inflammatory, anti-viral, and antibiotic properties, which are not destroyed during cooking, and their phytochemical compounds help to trigger healthy reactions within the body. Onions are also a good source of fiber and B vitamins. They have a multitude of culinary purposes!

Goji Berries

Goji berries may help to lower cholesterol levels and blood pressure.

Goji berries date back four thousand years. They are native to Asia, and have been used in Tibetan medicine as a tonic for the kidneys, cleansing the blood, eye conditions, skin rashes, and liver disease, along with other medicinal uses. Goji berries may help to lower cholesterol levels and blood pressure. Goji berries are a super-rich source of antioxidants, high in vitamin C, and a good source of calcium, potassium, iron, selenium, and zinc. Goji berries also contain B2 (riboflavin), as well as phytochemicals, beta carotene, polysaccharides, and zeaxanthin. Goji berries contain digestive inhibitors called lectins. However, soaking these berries in warm water for ten minutes before use can help reduce lectins, and also release important nutrients for bio-availability.

HERBS AND SPICES

Many of the aromatic spices, such as cinnamon, cloves, ginger, saffron, and cardamom, originated in Asia many centuries ago. At that time Arabs acted as the go-betweens for trading between Asia and Europe, until European explorers began traveling to India and other Asian lands to do their own trading. Spices were used not only to add flavor to dishes, but also for medicinal purposes, such as stimulating the appetite and aiding digestion. They vary in colors, textures, and flavors throughout the world, with each culture having its favorites and traditions. Spices are a wonderful way of adding small amounts of beneficial compounds to the diet.

Culinary herbs have also been around for centuries. A variety of different species are grown in many different parts of the world. Herbs were used in folklore, as trading commodities, for medicinal and botanical purposes, and later were used in cooking to add flavor to foods.

There are many different herbs and spices, and they all have their own important nutritional compounds. Here are some of my favorites:

❀ **Ginger** ~ Used very often in Indian and Asian cuisine, ginger has an intensely fragrant aroma and a spicy bite. Its natural oil, gingerol, is a powerful antioxidant and responsible for ginger's anti-inflammatory nature. It also helps the body to recover faster from exercise and ward off arthritis. Ginger helps to lower blood sugar, and may be beneficial to the cardiovascular system. Ginger also acts as a circulatory agent, is beneficial to the digestive system, and is a natural anti-nausea medication. Use in smoothies and juices, add grated or pressed to curries, soups, stir-frys and sauces, use in baking, or add to rice while cooking.

- **Garlic** ~ Known as a vegetable, herb, and spice, garlic contains a powerful medicinal compound called allicin, which also gives it an intensely enticing aroma. Garlic is a natural antibiotic with immune-enhancing properties. It helps prevent and treat fungal, bacterial, and parasitic infections, and has also shown cardiovascular and anti-tumor activity. Garlic is rich in manganese, B6, vitamin C, and selenium, and can enhance the flavor of just about any savory dish.
- **Cinnamon** ~ Like nutmeg, cinnamon was once a very valuable trade commodity. Today it is well known for its health benefits, and it is a warm and inviting spice reminiscent of the holidays. Cinnamon, with its very distinct flavor, regulates blood sugar and may help lower LDL cholesterol. It has anti-inflammatory and anti-carcinogenic properties, and is high in potassium, calcium, iron, magnesium, B6, and vitamins A and C. It also contains dietary fiber and protein. In addition, cinnamon is anti-viral and anti-fungal, freshens breath, helps keep gums healthy, and is a rich source of antioxidants.
- **Cloves** ~ Are native to the islands of Indonesia, and were another high-priced trading commodity

during the thirteenth and fourteenth centuries. Cloves strengthen the digestive system, decrease inflammation and pain, and protect the liver. Cloves help to stabilize blood sugar and boost immunity. Cloves are also a natural remedy for gum disease and can provide headache relief. They are super-high in potassium, calcium, magnesium, and iron, and are also a good source of B6, vitamin A, sodium, dietary fiber, and protein. Their rich, spicy flavor, makes them a great addition to baking savory and sweet dishes, hot and cold drinks, soups, and wholegrain breakfast bowls.

⊛ **Cayenne** ~ Its name comes from its place of origin, the Cayenne region of French Guiana, and it was first introduced to Europe by Christopher Columbus. Cayenne pepper has been used therapeutically and in cuisines all over the world. Cayenne pepper is a type of capsicum, and when used regularly in small amounts is said to have anti-cancer properties. It is a natural stimulant, and increases energy and metabolism. Cayenne pepper increases immunity, helps to clear respiratory and nasal congestion, and relieves flatulence. Cayenne is heart-strengthening and acts as a pain reliever. It is a rich source of vitamin A, vitamin B6, and vitamin C, as well as a good source of potassium, magnesium, iron, dietary fiber, and protein. This red-hot spice can be added to sauces, soups, and other savory dishes to give them a kick.

Cayenne pepper increases immunity, helps to clear respiratory and nasal congestion, and relieves flatulence.

⊛ **Turmeric** ~ Its medicinal uses date back thousands of years to Southeast Asia. A relative of the ginger family, turmeric's medicinal properties are similar to that of ginger. Because it is a natural anti-inflammatory, it has been used in Chinese medicine as a pain reliever and digestive aid. Turmeric's anti-inflammatory properties are also known to improve skin conditions, such as psoriasis and eczema, and help relieve joint-related conditions, such as arthritis. Turmeric is nutrient-dense in potassium, iron, magnesium, B6, and vitamin C, and is a good source of dietary fiber, protein, calcium, and sodium. Turmeric has a rich orange-yellow color and a bitter taste. Add turmeric to soups, sauces, rice and vegetable dishes, smoothies, and teas.

Basil ~ Is a member of the mint family and comes in different varieties and colors. The most common basil in the United States is the basil used in Mediterranean cuisine, found in pesto sauce, marinara sauce, and pizza toppings, along with other culinary purposes. Thai basil, holy basil, sweet basil, and lemon basil all originated in Asia and are used in Indian, Thai, and other Asian cuisines, and to flavor dishes such as stir frys, soups, and salads. Basil is a natural antiseptic, and is also known as an insect repellant. Some inedible varieties are grown in gardens specially to repel pests. Basil has been used for centuries to treat and reverse disease. In addition to being a rich source of vitamin A, vitamin C, calcium, magnesium, potassium, and iron, it has anti-inflammatory properties and is high in antioxidants, making it beneficial to cancer prevention and strengthening to the immune system. Basil is a great accompaniment to any tomato-based dish, soups and sauces, or as a topping on salads.

Basil is a natural antiseptic, and is also known as an insect repellant.

✿ **Parsley** ~ A vegetable, herb, and spice, and native to the central Mediterranean region. Parsley was once associated with death in Greece and England; old folklore believed that if parsley grew in an English garden, there would be a death within a year. Parsley is rich in vitamin K and vitamin C, along with a good amount of folate, vitamin A, and iron. It also contains volatile oils and flavonoids, whose compounds help stave off free radicals. In addition to boosting immunity and acting as an anti-inflammatory agent, parsley is also heart-healthy, due to its high concentration of vitamin K. Delicious in tabbouleh and added to soups, juices, and dressings.

✿ **Nutmeg** ~ Comes from a tropical evergreen tree native to Indonesia. Its seeds are ground into a very distinctive fragrant spice. Nutmeg is one of the rarest spices, and at one time was an extremely valuable commodity that nations would battle each other for. Only a small amount is needed to add delicious flavor to dishes, but that small amount packs a powerful nutritional punch. Nutmeg is rich in B vitamins, vitamin C, vitamin A, potassium, calcium, magnesium, iron, and zinc. Nutmeg is also known for its anti-fungal, anti-depressant, and digestive properties. Its oils have been used therapeutically as a pain reliever, helping to relieve toothaches, muscle aches, and joint aches. Sprinkle it on your breakfast grains and add it to baked goods and smoothies.

Nutmeg is also known for its anti-fungal, anti-depressant, and digestive properties.

✿ **Sage** ~ Is an herb and a spice, and comes from the mint family. Sage is indigenous to the

Mediterranean, and dates back to ancient Greek and Roman times. Sage was well known for its healing properties, and was also used as a preservative for other foods, due to its terpene antioxidants. As well as being a powerful source of vitamin K, calcium, iron and B6, it is a good source of vitamin A, magnesium, and vitamin C. Sage also contains dietary fiber and protein. Sage may help improve brain function, preventing cognitive decline. It contains antioxidant and anti-inflammatory properties, and helps to fight free-radical damage. It may also protect the heart from atherosclerosis, and help relieve lung conditions such as bronchial asthma. Sage contains flavonoids, and volatile oils which act as powerful antioxidants, strengthens immunity, and improves skin and bone health. The leaves have a deep green-grayish color with a strong, warm, earthy fragrance and taste. Add it to savory dishes, soups and sauces, and roasted vegetables.

PREPARING NUT AND SEED MILKS

Preparing your own nut and seed milks ensures that you are receiving all the nutrients from nut and seed superfoods, without the unnecessary fillers and preservatives that store-bought varieties tend to contain. It is always convenient to have store-bought nut and seed milks on hand when time is limited, but, whenever possible, taking time to prepare your own can have greater health benefits.

Best raw unsalted nuts to use:

- Walnuts
- Cashews
- Hazelnuts
- Almonds

- Macadamias
- Pecans
- Brazils

Best raw seeds to use:

- Hemp seeds
  (hemp seed milk
  does not need
  to be strained)

- Golden flaxseed

  Both of these seeds do
  not need to be soaked

What you will need:

- Super Blender,
  NutriBullet Rx,
  or Vitamix

- Nut milk
  strainer bag
- Milk jug

Tip: Nuts naturally contain phytic acid and enzyme inhibitors, which can irritate the digestive system and even lead to nutrient deficiencies over time. Soaking your nuts prior to consumption breaks down phytic acid and neutralizes the enzyme inhibitors. Soaking your nuts also increases the bioavailability of the nutrients and important enzymes that increase the absorption of these nutrients.

Directions

1. Soak 1 cup of nuts by covering them until they are submerged with filtered water and a ¼ teaspoon of ground Himalayan pink sea salt. Raw seeds such as pumpkin and sunflower can also be soaked using this method.

2. Leave on the counter covered overnight or refrigerated. This will plump up the nuts and make them easier to digest.

3. In the morning rinse the nuts well with filtered water.

4. Add 1 cup of nuts to your blender with 5 cups of filtered water. If you prefer a vanilla flavor, add 1 teaspoon of vanilla extract. If you prefer it a little sweet, add 1 tablespoon of coconut nectar or agave.

5. Blend until smooth and milky, then pour through your milk strainer bag into your milk jug, cover, and store in your refrigerator for 3–5 days. If you like, you can make smaller amounts of different milks so you are not consuming the same milk every day. Make sure you wash your strainer bag well and sterilize it in hot water after every use.

Walnuts

These nuts are rich in essential fatty acids (omega-3 fatty acids in particular), which are not so easy to find in the plant kingdom. Omega-3 fatty acids decrease inflammation in the body, enhance mood, and increase focus. Known as the brain food, the nut itself even resembles the cerebral cortex of the brain. This powerhouse is rich in magnesium, iron, potassium, phosphorous, calcium, selenium, and B vitamins, especially B6, with a modest mix of vitamins A, C, E and K. Walnuts are also high in fiber and protein.

Cashews

The cashew may be the best tasting nut, adding a smooth, creamy flavor and texture to many recipes. Cashews are high in monounsaturated and polyunsaturated fats, provide a good source of protein, and are rich in potassium, phosphorous, manganese, copper, selenium, iron, and B6.

Hazelnuts

Hazelnuts are rich in antioxidants, and boost brain function. They are delicious, especially when roasted or toasted. They are rich in vitamin E, manganese, copper, and thiamine, which helps give the metabolism a boost. They are also a good source of folate, B6, and iron, with over 4 grams of protein and almost 3 grams of fiber per ounce.

Almonds

Almonds are actually the seeds of the fruit of the almond tree, and are the most popular nut and nut milk choice, with good reason. Almonds are a rich source of vitamin E, calcium, magnesium, and iron, as well as a good source of selenium, niacin, copper, and zinc. They also help keep bones strong, reduce inflammation, boost metabolism, and help regulate blood pressure.

Macadamias

Macadamias are a rich source of Vitamin A, iron, protein, thiamin, riboflavin, niacin, and folate. They are full of antioxidants, and may be beneficial to heart health. I love the creamy, buttery taste and texture of this nut. Probably my favorite nut milk, and perfect for making my fruit and nut-cream toppings for puddings and breakfast bowls.

Pecans

Pecans are a great source of magnesium, potassium, iron, and fiber, as well as a good source of monounsaturated fats, polyunsaturated fats, and calcium. When you think of pecans, you probably think of pecan pie, but that is not all they are good for. Apart from making nut milk, they are also delicious roasted or toasted, and topped on breakfast bowls and salads.

Brazils

Brazils are a large nut with a crunchy texture and a creamy flavor. They are a rich source of magnesium, potassium, calcium, and iron, and a great source of protein and fiber. Brazils are heart healthy! Enjoy them in a nut milk, in my superfood bars, or in a smoothie.

Hemp Seeds

Hemp seeds are on my list of superfoods. They are easily digested and a great source of plant protein. They are a complete protein, containing all eight essential amino acids, which is why they not only make a perfect plant milk, but are great added to smoothies and drinks to increase protein content. Hemp seeds are a rich source of essential fatty acids and a good source of magnesium, sulfur, calcium, vitamin E, phosphorus, potassium, sodium, iron, and zinc.

Flaxseeds

Flaxseeds, also known as linseeds, are rich in omega-3 fatty acids. Golden flaxseeds are a little higher in nutritional value than regular flaxseeds. Flax milk has a creamy texture with a slightly nutty flavor, and is a good source of protein, magnesium, iron, calcium, and B6. In addition to making a great plant milk, flaxseeds can be ground down and added to smoothies, wholegrain cereals, breads, muffins, and burgers.

PHYTIC ACID

Phytic acid is a digestive inhibitor found in protein-rich foods such as grains, beans, legumes, nuts, and seeds in varying amounts, and in much lesser amounts in root vegetables and tubers. Phytic acid, also known as phytate, is an anti-nutrient because it interferes with the absorption of important minerals such as calcium, iron, and zinc, and can possibly lead to a deficiency of one or more of those minerals over time. However, a mineral deficiency is much less likely when consuming a well-balanced, vitamin C-rich, whole food, plant-based diet. There is a lot of confusing information regarding phytic acid, and its role in causing digestive problems attributed to certain types of foods. I do not think is a good idea to eliminate grains, beans/lugumes, nuts, and seeds from the diet for fear of phytic acid. Choosing to eat animal protein over these important nutrient-rich, plant-based foods is far more detrimental to health.

If you are concerned that foods such as grains, beans/legumes, etc., may adversely affect your digestive system, following are some methods that can greatly reduce the amount of phytic acid found in these foods and, thereby, reduce digestive system upset.

Soaking ~ Soaking is important for harder grains such as kamut, spelt, and wheat berries. Harder grains should be soaked in water for 12 hours. Buckwheat, millet, and brown rice only require 8 hours. Use filtered water and you can also add a little apple cider vinegar to grains, about a tablespoon per cup of water. You only need enough water to submerge the grains. Make sure to keep them covered. It is not necessary to rinse them, but you can. If you do not want to rinse them before cooking, make sure you soak the grains in the required amount of water or vegetable broth for cooking. (See "Cooking Your Grains" in this book).

Soak beans up to 12 hours. When soaking beans, add enough water to submerge all beans. For smaller beans, such as black beans, use 1 tbsp. apple cider vinegar per cup of water, and for larger beans such as kidney beans add a ¼ tsp. baking soda, changing baking soda water a couple of times during the soaking period if your schedule allows. Rinse beans well when soaking time is up. Grains and beans also tend to cook faster when presoaked. Soaking beans helps break down/neutralize phytic acid, making the important nutrients they contain more bioavailable.

Grinding ~ I like to grind grains such as oats and buckwheat, to make my own flours. Millet, teff, and quinoa can also be ground to make flour, but toast these grains in a dry skillet before grinding. You can also use the soaking method for flours (rinsing is not required when soaking flours). Cover and soak overnight. Use in a recipe the next day. Regarding soaking nuts, please see my section on making nut milks.

Roasting ~ Roasting nuts does not require soaking first. Roasting nuts also breaks down phytic acid, releases their natural oils, and enhances their flavor, making them taste even more delicious. Just make sure the nuts you use are raw and unsalted. Preheat oven to 300–350°F. Line a baking sheet with unbleached parchment paper (or forgo the parchment paper, and use a non-stick baking sheet) and spread nuts out evenly. Roast for 8–10 minutes (pine nuts take just 5 minutes), or toast them on the stovetop using a dry skillet. Move them around during cooking so they do not burn.

Sprouting ~ Sprouting is another method, more superior to soaking. Sprouted grains, beans, nuts, and seeds have a very high nutrient content and they become much easier to digest. You can also purchase them already sprouted. If you cannot find them already sprouted in the grocery store, you can purchase them online.

Fermenting ~ Fermenting grains and beans also breaks down phytic acid and releases nutrients. Sourdough bread is made by the fermentation of dough using a naturally occurring probiotic such as lactobacilli mixed with yeast. Miso, tamari sauce, and tempeh are fermented soybeans.

Healing the Gut with a Whole Food, Plant-Based Lifestyle

Prebiotics and probiotics both serve vital roles in the health of the human gut. Probiotics are good bacteria that reside naturally in the gastrointestinal tract, keeping it healthy, clean, and functioning optimally. To work efficiently, these probiotics need to be fed a health-sustaining diet of prebiotics, which are made up of un-digestible forms of fiber found in plant foods.

A diet high in animal protein and processed foods is detrimental to healthy intestinal bacteria (probiotics). Foods high in animal protein and processed foods increase the amount of acid buildup in the body, disrupting pH levels and harboring unhealthy bacteria growth. Unhealthy bacteria disrupt the work of the probiotics (good bacteria) by taking over residency within the gastrointestinal tract. The unhealthy bacteria then provide a perfect environment for damaging viruses, yeast infections, and scavenging parasites to manifest. This environment depletes the healthy intestinal flora/bacteria while the unhealthy flora/bacteria continue to multiply.

When a nutrient-dense, plant-based diet is consumed, the body becomes more alkaline, pH levels become healthy, and prebiotics begin to increase through the consumption of different forms of fiber found in plant foods such as: raw and cooked garlic, raw and cooked onions, raw and cooked leeks, bananas, raw asparagus, raw chicory root, raw dandelion greens, raw Jerusalem artichoke, barley, oats, apples, cacao, aloe vera, flaxseeds, and seaweeds. These prebiotic foods feed the probiotics found in the gut, allowing beneficial intestinal flora/bacteria to flourish. Prebiotics provide the nourishment for good bacteria (probiotics) already living in the gut. A probiotic is a live microorganism found naturally in the body that can also be consumed through the intake of plant foods such as: sauerkraut, kimchi, sour pickles, miso, tempeh, sourdough bread, kombucha, and olives.

When a nutrient-dense, plant-based diet is consumed, the body becomes more alkaline . . .

SUPPLEMENTS

Store shelves and online sites are overloaded with seemingly endless varieties and combinations of supplements, accompanied by claims of a plethora of health benefits. But, seriously, why would you want to put a processed, isolated nutrient into your body when you can obtain the real thing from whole plant foods? Good health is a result of eating whole plant foods that provide proper nutrition, and should not come from powdered, encapsulated, gelatin-covered, processed, isolated compounds. Makes perfect sense doesn't it?

Then why are so many people convinced that they need to bombard their bodies with concentrated and sometimes inappropriate quantities of these substances? Unfortunately, in our society today, people become so extensively stressed that it affects the digestive system, compelling most overly busy people to seek a quick fix through pills, supplements, and unnatural derivatives of foods. Optimal health should always begin with whole food nutrition first; that is, foods in their natural state with minimal processing, such as fruits, vegetables, legumes, whole grains, nuts, and seeds, along with lifestyle changes including stress-reducing practices. Try not to be fooled by highly marketed, so-called new wonder trends.

A couple of the latest, highly marketed, wonder trends are the animal collagen craze and the seemingly ubiquitous animal-bone broth craze. Most of you are aware that the majority of cattle raised today are fattened up with synthetic hormones, fed genetically modified corn, and housed in cramped, close quarters, most of the time never having access to the outdoors. This unhealthy environment makes them highly susceptible to disease. Why would we want to consume these poor, decaying animals, and drink broth make from their bones? These animals have also been shown to be susceptible to lead exposure through feed and

Optimal health should always begin with whole food nutrition first . . .

through contaminates when pasture raised. Animals that do not show clinical signs of toxic lead exposure are not routinely tested. This lead accumulates in the bones and, therefore, ends up in bone broth. I believe bone broth to be more harmful than healthy. A diet rich in plants actually offers a higher source of collagen building blocks than animal collagen and bone broth. Furthermore, plants are much higher in nutrient density.

It is important to have regular blood work and to check B12 and vitamin D levels. B12 is the one supplement I would recommend that you take if you are vegan. Make sure the B12 supplement you choose comes from a vegan source and does not contain any foods that you know you have a sensitivity to. Also, if you know that your body requires a particular supplement, or if you are found to be deficient in a certain nutrient, you can then supplement. Furthermore, if you are taking certain prescription drugs that you know deplete certain nutrients, then supplementation may also be necessary. However, as for taking a synthetic multivitamin just in case, how about consuming a whole food, plant-based diet just in case!

A diet rich in plants actually offers a higher source of collagen building blocks than animal collagen and bone broth.

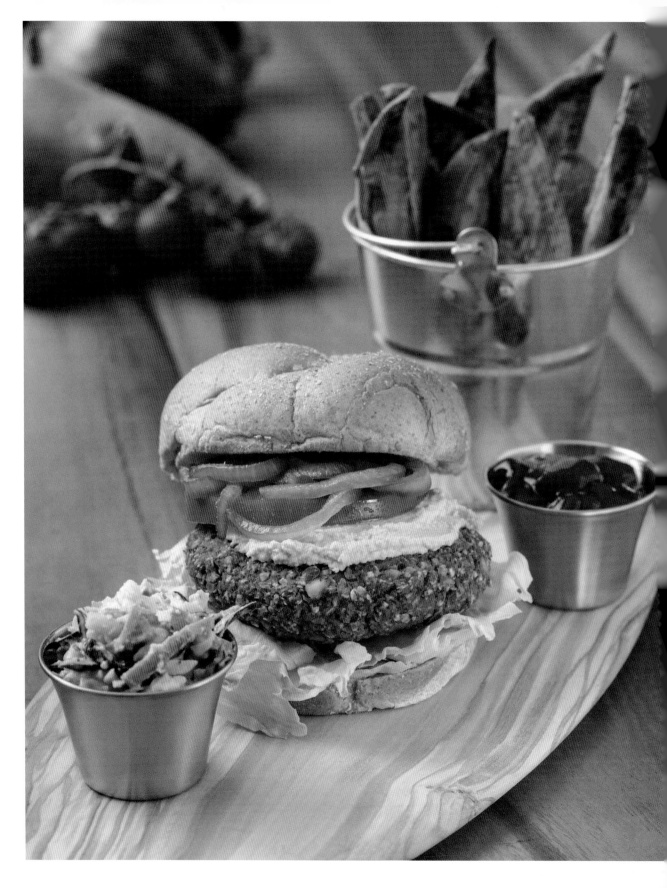

Part Two

Recipes

Live Simply Plant Based recipes are packed full of nutrients to ensure that you will receive a well-balanced, whole food, plant-based diet. All the recipes are 100 percent vegan and gluten-free. They are simple and easy to follow to make your transition smooth and enjoyable. From liquid nutrition, feeding your body at the cellular level, to high-energy breakfast bowls to begin your day with super nutrition, you will find everything you need to transition to optimal health. The main dishes are a combination of raw foods and cooked foods, and all the dishes contain plenty of plant proteins and complex carbohydrates to ensure that your body is well fueled. These foods are easily digested and the fiber assists in keeping blood-sugar levels stable and energy levels high.

There is a section on dressings, sauces, and toppings so you can make your own instead of using store purchased, processed varieties. I have made the recipes quick and easy to follow, as I realize we all have time constraints. In my snack section, you will find some delicious and nutritious options, again with easy-to-follow instructions. This is the way I eat, this is my lifestyle and it works! The repeat of some of the ingredients is purposeful, as these ingredients are always readily available in your local supermarket and easy to prepare. I hope you have fun with the recipes, and enjoy all the different flavors and textures.

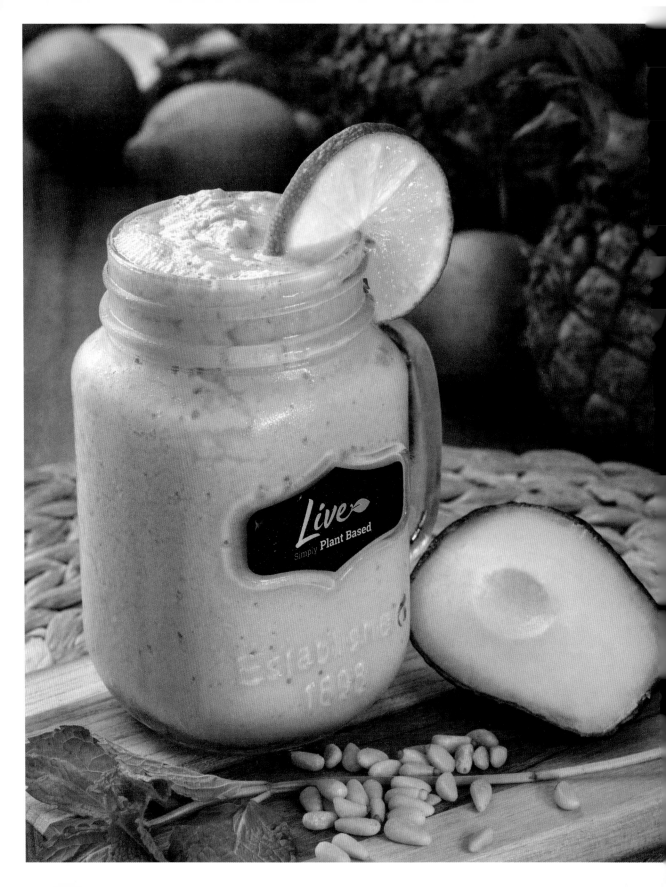

Liquid Nutrition

Smoothies and juices are a quick and easy way to fuel the body on the go. Fresh juice fuels our bodies at the cellular level. Juicing alkalizes the body, cleansing and cleaning it from the inside out. Juicing provides for an immediate absorption of nutrients that you can feel right after you have consumed it! You will notice that I use a lot of lemons and limes in my juices, because they are loaded with vitamin C, which not only boosts immunity, but also helps to increase the absorption of nutrients from other foods. Smoothies and juices are great as a quick breakfast on the go. If you are trying to gain weight, maybe have one along with a whole-grain breakfast (see my high-energy breakfast recipes).

There are some who argue that smoothies can contain as much sugar as a soft drink, due to their high fruit content. Think about it: a smoothie contains a lot more than just fruit sugar, it is loaded with antioxidants (free radical eradicators). My smoothies and juices can all be prepared in a super blender, Vitamix, or NutriBullet RX.

For any recipes containing nut or seed milks, if you choose to make you own over store bought varieties, please find instructions on preparing nut and seed milks on pages 74–76.

Tip: My juices that end with the word "recovery" are formulated to be especially effective as post-exercise recovery drinks. They are light and fresh, alkaline, and higher in carbohydrates than protein. This makes them perfect for exercise recovery and boosting energy, and they provide easy assimilation and digestibility.

Joint Mover Recovery

1 cup hemp or almond milk
½ cup frozen pineapple or
	mango chunks
1 fresh banana
½ tsp. turmeric
½ tsp. cinnamon
½ tsp. ginger
1 tbsp. raw unsalted cashews
½ tsp. maca powder (optional)
1 medjool date, pitted

Green Protein

1 cup almond milk
1 tsp. spirulina powder
1 tbsp. almond butter
1 fresh banana
1 tsp. chia seeds
1 medjool date, pitted

Choco Potion

1 cup almond milk
1 fresh banana
½ tsp. maca powder
½ tsp. raw cacao powder
1 tbsp. raw almond butter
1 medjool date, pitted

Sweet Spirulina Recovery

½ cup hemp milk
½ cup coconut water
½ banana
2 tbsp. hemp seeds
1 heaping tsp. raw cashew
	butter
½ tsp. spirulina
1 tbsp. goji berries
1 medjool date, pitted

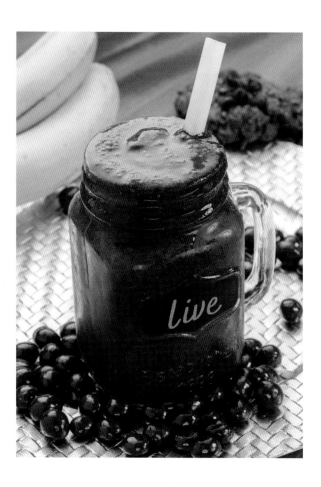

Avocado Dream

1 cup coconut water
1 small avocado
½ cup frozen pineapple chunks
1 lime, juiced
¼ cup fresh mint leaves
1 tbsp. pine nuts
1 chunk fresh aloe, peeled and
    rinsed (optional)
Thick and creamy.

Green Oatmeal

1 cup almond milk
2 tbsp. gluten-free oats
1 medjool date, pitted
1 handful fresh spinach leaves
1 fresh or frozen banana
2 tbsp. hemp seeds
½ tsp. maca powder

Spinach Kale Surprise

1 cup coconut water
1 handful fresh spinach leaves
1 handful fresh kale, stalks
    removed
1 apple cored and quartered
½ cup frozen pineapple chunks

Brown Rice Blend

1 cup almond milk
½ cup cooked brown rice or 2 tbsp.
    brown rice protein powder
1 banana
1 tbsp. goji berries
1 medjool date, pitted
1 tbsp. raw, unsalted cashews
½ tsp. maca powder

Digestive Boost Recovery

1 cup water or coconut water
½ cup ice
½ frozen banana
½ small papaya
½ cup frozen pineapple chunks
¼ tsp. matcha green tea
3 tbsp. hemp seeds
1 medjool date, pitted
1 small chunk fresh aloe, peeled
    and rinsed (optional)

Iced Green Tea Latte

½ cup coconut or hemp milk
½ cup coconut water
1 tsp. matcha green tea powder
1 medjool date, pitted
½ cup ice

Thick and Creamy

½ cup frozen pineapple chunks
Zest of 1 lime
1 lime juiced
½ cup coconut water
1 tbsp. soaked sunflower seeds
    (optional)
½ avocado
Thick and creamy, I like to eat it
    with a spoon.

Strawberry Ginger Recovery

½ banana
½ cup frozen strawberries
1 tsp. grated ginger root
1 small chunk fresh aloe vera
    (optional)
1 cup almond milk
3 tbsp. hemp seeds
1 medjool date, pitted

Tip: For a refreshing energizer/
recovery, use coconut water instead of
almond milk, only 2 tbsp. hemp seeds,
and add ¼ tsp. maca powder.

Wake Me Up Recovery

1 cup coconut water
1 tsp. grated ginger root
½ cup frozen mango
½ banana
2 tbsp. hemp seeds
¼ tsp. matcha green tea powder
1 small chunk of fresh aloe vera or ¼
    cup aloe juice (optional)

Morning Refresher Recovery

1 cup coconut water
½ cup frozen mango chunks
½ cup blueberries
1 tsp. grated ginger root
1 medjool date, pitted
2 tbsp. hemp seeds

Morning Energizer Recovery

1 pear, halved and cored
1 tsp. grated ginger root
½ cup frozen mango
Zest from one lemon
1 lemon, juiced
1 medjool date, pitted
1 cup coconut water
2 tbsp. hemp seeds

Best Re-Hydrator Recovery

1 cup coconut water
Zest from 1 lemon
½ lemon, juiced
Pinch ground Himalayan pink sea salt
1 medjool date, pitted
2 tbsp. hemp seeds
1 small chunk fresh aloe vera, peeled
    and rinsed, or ¼ cup aloe juice
    (optional)

Tip: As a morning energizer, add
¼ tsp. matcha green tea powder.

Morning Energy Burst Recovery

1 cup of coconut water
½ cup frozen blueberries
Zest of 1 lemon
1 lemon juiced
1 small chunk of fresh aloe
    peeled and rinsed or ¼ cup
    aloe juice (optional)
3 tbsp. hemp seeds
¼ tsp. matcha green tea powder
1 medjool date, pitted

Brain Boost Recovery

1 cup walnut milk
1 medjool date, pitted
1 small banana
⅓ cup frozen mango
2 tbsp. hemp seeds
¼ tsp. maca

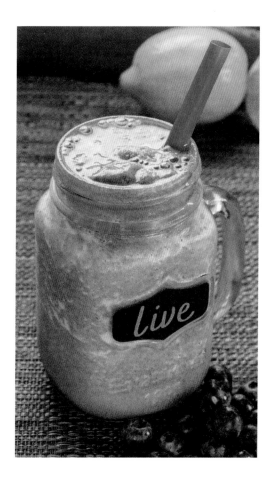

Digestive Refresher Recovery

1 cup water or coconut water
Zest of 1 lemon
1 lemon juiced
2 medjool dates, pitted
3 tbsp. hemp seeds
1 cup frozen papaya
1 small chunk fresh aloe

Super Spirulina Recovery

1 cup walnut milk or other
    plant milk
½ frozen banana
1 tbsp. chia seeds
1 tsp. spirulina powder
1 tbsp. raw, sprouted, unsalted
    pumpkin seed butter
1 tsp. coconut nectar or 2
    medjool dates, pitted

Green Mango

1 cup coconut water
1 lime juiced
½ cup frozen mango
½ avocado
2 tbsp. hemp seeds
1 medjool date, pitted

Green Recovery

1 cup almond milk
1 banana
⅓ cup frozen blueberries
½ tsp. chlorella
½ tsp. spirulina
2 tbsp. sprouted pumpkin seeds
1 tbsp. hemp seeds

Body Cleanser

1 cup water
1 cup coconut water
1 handful parsley
1 lime, juiced
1 lemon, juiced
½ cucumber, cut into chunks
1 apple, cored and quartered

Carrot Ginger

1 cup coconut water
1 cup water or ice
2 carrots, peeled and quartered
1 handful fresh parsley
1 apple, cored and quartered
1 small chunk peeled ginger
1 lemon juiced

Light and Fresh

1 cup seedless watermelon
½ cup frozen strawberries
1 cup coconut water
Zest of 1 lime
1 lime, juiced
1 medjool date, pitted

Clean Kick

1 cup coconut water
½ cup water
1 cup ice
1 cup arugula
1 cup spring mix
1 large lemon, juiced
1 lime, juiced
½ avocado
1 small chunk fresh turmeric,
    peeled, or ½ tsp. powder
1 medjool date, pitted
⅓ cup frozen mango
1 tbsp. hemp seeds

Sour Citrus Cleanse Recovery

1 orange, juiced
1 lime, juiced

1 lemon, juiced
½ tsp. chlorella powder
2 tbsp. hemp seeds
½ cup coconut water
¼ cup aloe juice or 1 small
    chunk fresh aloe vera, peeled
    and rinsed

Green Banana Citrus Cleanse Recovery

1 lemon, juiced
1 lime, juiced
1 cup coconut water
½ tsp. chlorella
½ tsp. spirulina
1 banana
2 tbsp. hemp seeds
1 medjool date, pitted

Black Cherry Citrus Boost Recovery

1 cup coconut water
½ cup frozen black cherries
Zest of 1 lemon
1 lemon, juiced
1 lime, juiced
3 tbsp. hemp seeds
½ tsp. chlorella powder

Banana Lime Recovery

Juice of 1 lime
¾ cup alkaline water or coconut water
⅓ cup ice
1 banana
2 tbsp. freshly ground golden flaxseed
2 tbsp. hemp seeds
½ tsp. maca
1 medjool date, pitted, or 1 tsp. agave

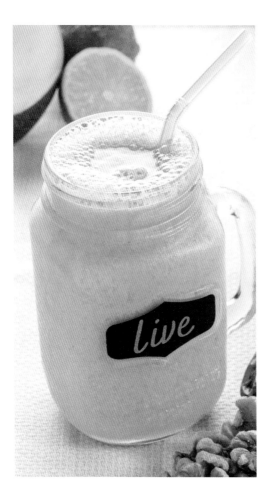

Chlorella Avocado Mint Mango

1 cup water
½ tsp. chlorella
½ avocado
½ cup fresh mint leaves
½ cup frozen mango
2 medjool dated, pitted
3 tbsp. hemp seeds

Matcha Açaí Energy Recovery

1 cup coconut water
½ banana
⅓ cup frozen mango chunks
3 tbsp. hemp seeds
½ tsp. matcha green tea powder
½ tsp. açaí powder
1 medjool date, pitted

Energizing Digestion Tamer

1 cup coconut water
½ cup frozen papaya chunks
⅓ cup frozen black cherries
1 small chunk fresh ginger,
    peeled

1 small chunk fresh aloe vera,
    peeled and rinsed
2 tbsp. hemp seeds
1 medjool date, pitted
½ tsp. matcha green tea powder

Matcha Berry Citrus Burst Recovery

1 cup coconut water
½ cup frozen mixed berries
Zest from 1 large lemon or 2
    small
1 large lemon, juiced, or 2 small
1 small chunk fresh aloe vera or
    ¼ cup aloe vera juice
2 tbsp. hemp seeds
½ tsp. matcha green tea powder

Hemp Papaya Recovery

1 cup hemp milk
3 tbsp hemp seed
½ cup frozen papaya
zest of 1 lime
1 lime, juiced
½ banana
1 medjool date, pitted
⅓ cup strawberries
⅓ cup frozen blueberries
½ tsp. maca powder

Green Apple Chlorella Recovery

1 cup coconut water
1 Granny Smith apple, cored and
    quartered
Zest and juice from 1 lemon
Zest and juice from 1 lime
2 tbsp. hemp seeds
½ frozen banana
1 chunk fresh aloe vera or ¼ cup
    aloe vera juice (optional)
½ tsp. chlorella powder
1 medjool date, pitted

Spirulina Shake

1 cup macadamia nut milk or
    other plant milk
½ cup frozen strawberries
½ cup frozen mango
2 Medjool dates, pitted
½ tsp. spirulina
½ tsp. coconut shreds
1 tsp. soaked (10 minutes in warm
    water) goji berries, drained and
    rinsed
Place all ingredients in blender except
    coconut and goji berries, use them
    for topping.

Avocado Grape

1 cup coconut water
½ avocado
1 cup green seedless grapes
½ frozen banana
Juice of 1 lemon
Juice of 1 lime
1 tbsp. hemp seeds
½ tsp. maca powder

Smooth Move

1 cup water or coconut water
Zest and juice of 1 lemon
½ cup frozen strawberries
4 prunes
2 tbsp. hemp seeds
1 tsp. açaí powder
1 chunk fresh aloe vera or ¼ cup
    aloe juice

Orange Tahini Recovery Smoothie

2 oranges, juiced
1 tbsp. tahini cream (see Tip on
    page 134)
1 tbsp. hemp protein or 2 tbsp.
    hemp seeds
½ tsp. matcha green tea powder
½ frozen banana

⅓ cup frozen strawberries
1 cup water

Digestive Soother

1 cup cooled licorice root tea
½ cup coconut water
1 small chunk peeled fresh ginger
Juice of 1 lemon
2 tbsp. hemp seeds
1 medjool date, pitted
1 small chunk fresh aloe vera or
    ¼ cup aloe juice (optional)

Watercress Cleanse Recovery

1 cup watercress
Juice of 1 lime
Juice of 1 lemon
½ cup frozen pineapple
½ tsp. maca
2 tbsp. hemp seeds
1 medjool date, pitted
1 cup water

Simple Morning Cleanse

Juice of 1 or 2 lemons
½ cup boiling water
½ cup filtered water

Dragon Fruit Recovery

1 cup coconut water
1 medjool date, pitted
3 tbsp. hemp seeds
½ dragon fruit or 1 tsp. powder
½ banana
Juice of 1 lime
¼ cup frozen blueberries
¼ cup frozen strawberries

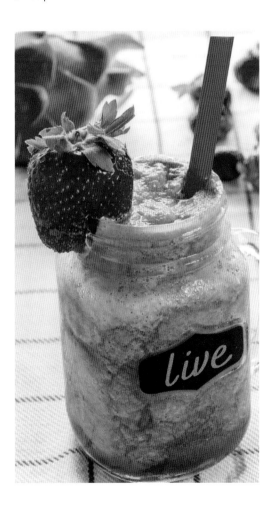

Pumpkin Mango Recovery

1 banana
½ cup pumpkin puree
½ tsp. maca
¾ cup hemp milk
½ tsp. allspice
½ cup frozen mango
1 tbsp. tahini
1 medjool date

Moringa Focus Recovery

1 cup coconut water
Juice of 1 lime
1 banana
½ cup frozen mango
1 tbsp. hemp protein or 3 tbsp.
    hemp seeds
1 medjool date, pitted
1 tsp. moringa

Watercress Recovery

1 cup coconut water
1 cup watercress
1 banana
Juice of 1 lime
2 tbsp. hemp seeds
1 medjool date, pitted
½ tsp. maca

Matcha Mango Recovery

1 cup coconut water
2 tbsp. hemp seeds
1 cup frozen mango chunks
1 chunk fresh aloe (inner fillet)
1 medjool date, pitted
½ tsp. matcha green tea powder
Zest and juice of 1 lime
¼ cup soaked cashews

Parsley Mint Recovery

1 cup coconut water
1 cup fresh parsley, stalks removed
½ cup fresh mint, stalks removed
Juice of 1 lemon
½ frozen banana
1 medjool date, pitted
2 tbsp. hemp seeds

Chlorella Lemon Berry Recovery

I cup water or coconut water
½ cup frozen strawberries
½ cup frozen blueberries
1 tsp. chlorella powder
3 tbsp. hemp seeds
Juice of 1 lemon
½ banana

½ cup ice
1 medjool date pitted (optional)
1 chunk fresh aloe peeled and
    rinsed (optional)

Spinach Mango Recovery

1 cup water or coconut water
2 cups baby spinach
½ tsp. chlorella
3 tbsp. hemp seeds
Juice of 1 orange
1 cup frozen mango
½ cup ice
1 chunk fresh aloe peeled and
    rinsed (optional)
1 medjool date, pitted

Here is my favorite juice extraction.
You will need a juicer for this, but I can
assure you that it will be well worth it!

Carrot Citrus Cleanse

6 large carrots
6 stalks of celery
1 apple, halved
1 large handful parsley
1 chunk ginger
Juice of 1 lemon
Juice of 1 lime

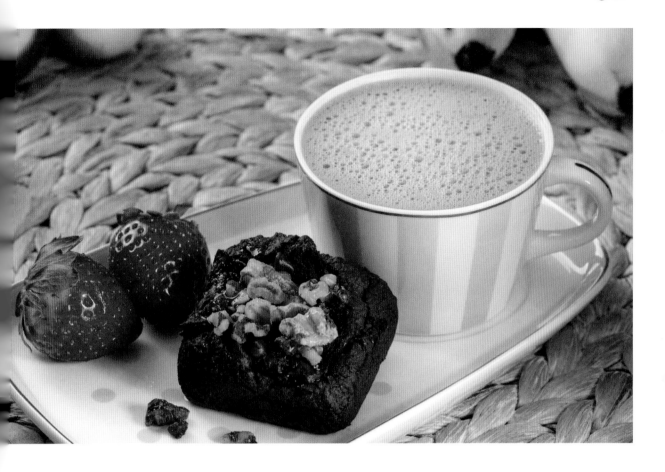

Matcha Green Tea Latte

1 cup cashew milk
1 tsp. matcha green tea powder
1 tsp. coconut palm sugar (optional)

Directions

1. Bring cashew milk to gentle boil on stovetop.

2. Place matcha green tea powder in a cup, gently whisk in hot cashew milk until frothy, and well blended. Add coconut palm sugar if desired. Serves 1.

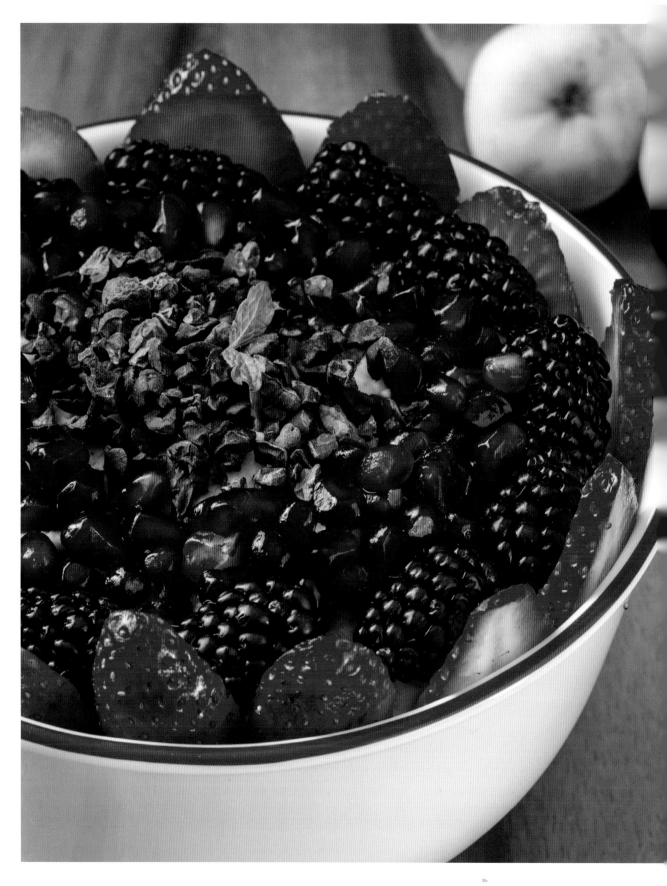

High-Energy Breakfasts

Whole grains are a great way to start your day! Packed full of energy-boosting B vitamins, whole grains help keep you feeling fuller longer. They stabilize blood sugar, help reduce cholesterol, lower the risk of type 2 diabetes, and reduce the risk of many colon-related diseases. I realize that with a busy schedule, it is easy to just grab the same box of cereal every day, which may be fine on occasion, as long as you choose a cereal that contains whole grains and is minimally processed, with no more than 5 grams of added sugar per ½ cup serving. However, taking a little extra time to prepare your breakfast in the morning will ensure that you are varying your diet and can increase your nutrient intake substantially.

I like to soak my grains in plant milk overnight before breakfast. Soaking will increase digestibility and speed up cooking time. The recipes below are for un-soaked grains. However, if you soak your grains, you can generally cut a few minutes off the cooking time. Try to vary your nut milks to avoid sensitivities. Hemp seed milk is very easily digested and fine to use on a regular basis. If you are preparing your own nut and seed milks please see page 74–76 for directions. If you are making your own rice milk see Tip on page 57, and if you are making your own oat milk see Tip on page 116.

Below are some recipes for my favorite breakfast grains. I hope you enjoy them as much as I do!

Teff Parfait

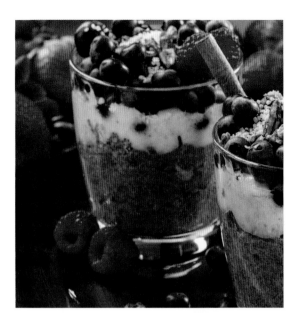

2 cups hemp milk
  (see seed milk recipe)

⅔ cup teff

1 unsweetened coconut yogurt

1 banana

½ cup blueberries

¼ cup raw unsalted walnuts

¼ cup raspberries

2 tsp. hemp seeds

2 cinnamon sticks

⅛ tsp. pink Himalayan pink salt

2 tsp. coconut nectar (optional)

Directions

1. Preheat oven 350°F. Spread walnuts out on a baking sheet and roast for 8–10 minutes and set aside.

2. Heat hemp milk and teff on stovetop to a slight boil, reduce to simmer, and cook for 15 minutes. Add salt just before cooking ends.

3. Place yogurt and banana in a food processor and pulse until smooth.

4. Divide teff into 2 short wide glasses, and top with yogurt banana cream, blueberries, walnuts, hemp seeds, raspberries and cinnamon sticks. Serves 2.

Almond Buckwheat

1 cup almond milk (see
   nut milk recipe)

⅓ cup buckwheat

¼ cup sliced fresh strawberries

½ tsp. chia seeds

¼ tsp. nutmeg

Pinch ground Himalayan
   sea salt (optional)

Directions

1. Bring almond milk to a
   slight boil and whisk in
   buckwheat. Lower to
   simmer and cook for 10
   minutes. Add salt just
   before cooking ends.

2. Place in a bowl and top
   with chia, strawberries, and
   nutmeg. Serves 1.

Almond Amaranth

1 cup almond milk (see
   nut milk recipe)

⅓ cup amaranth

⅓ cup sliced black
   seedless grapes

⅛ tsp. nutmeg

½ tsp. coconut nectar

Pinch ground Himalayan
   pink sea salt

Directions

1. Place almond milk and
   amaranth in a saucepan
   and bring to a slight boil,
   reduce to simmer, and
   cook for 25 minutes. Add
   salt before cooking ends.

2. Place in a bowl and top
   with sliced black grapes and
   nutmeg and drizzle with
   coconut nectar. Serves 1.

Goldenberry Oatmeal

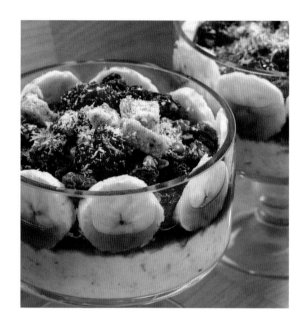

1 cup hemp milk
   (see seed milk recipe)

⅓ cup gluten-free steel-cut oats

⅓ cup goldenberries

¼ cup sprouted pumpkin seeds

1 banana

1 tsp. coconut nectar

⅛ tsp. Himalayan pink salt

⅛ tsp. ground ginger

⅛ tsp. ground turmeric

Directions

3.   Bring hemp milk to a slight boil, stir in oats,
     reduce to simmer, and cook for 10 minutes,
     add salt just before cooking ends.

4.   Transfer to a bowl, and top with goldenberries, banana,
     ginger, turmeric and coconut nectar. Serves 1.

Amaranth Bowl

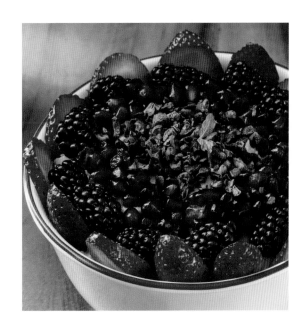

1 cup cashew milk
   (see nut milk recipe)

⅓ cup amaranth

½ cup sliced strawberries

⅓ cup blackberries

¼ cup pomegranate seeds

1 tbsp. cacao nibs

1 tsp. coconut nectar

⅛ tsp. pink Himalayan sea salt

Directions

1. Place cashew milk and amaranth in a saucepan, bring to a slight boil, reduce to simmer, and cook for 25 minutes. Add salt just before cooking ends.

2. Place in a bowl and top with strawberries, blackberries, pomegranate seeds, cacao nibs and coconut nectar. Serves 1.

Joint Mover
Teff Bowl

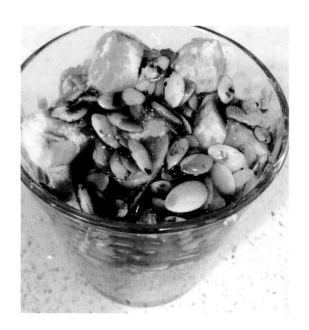

1 cup hemp milk (see
   seed milk recipe)

⅓ cup teff

⅛ tsp. Himalayan pink salt

1 banana

¼ cup sprouted pumpkin seeds

½ tsp. turmeric

¼ tsp. ginger

1 tsp. coconut nectar

Directions

1. Heat milk and teff to a slight boil, reduce to simmer and
   cook for 15 minutes, add salt just before cooking ends.

2. Transfer to a bowl and top with banana, pumpkin seeds,
   turmeric, ginger and coconut nectar. Serves 1.

Hemp Blackberry Buckwheat

1 cup hemp milk (see seed milk recipe)

⅓ cup buckwheat

½ banana, sliced

⅓ cup blackberries

2 hemp heart bites, finely diced (see resources)

2 tbsp. coconut yogurt

1 tbsp. chopped toasted walnuts (see toasting/roasting nuts)

1 tsp. coconut nectar

⅛ tsp. nutmeg

⅛ tsp. ground Himalayan pink sea salt

Directions

1. Bring hemp milk to a slight boil, stir in buckwheat,
    reduce to simmer and cook for 10 minutes.
    Add salt just before cooking ends.

2. Place cooked buckwheat in a bowl and top with
    banana, coconut yogurt, blackberries, toasted walnuts,
    hemp hearts, coconut nectar, and nutmeg. Serves 1.

Macadamia Oatmeal

1 cup macadamia nut milk (see nut milk recipe)

⅓ cup gluten-free steel-cut oats

2 tbsp. unsweetened applesauce

¼ tsp. cinnamon

¼ cup fresh blackberries

Pinch ground Himalayan pink sea salt

Directions

1. Bring macadamia milk to a slight boil and whisk in oats. Lower to simmer and cook for 10 minutes. Add salt just before cooking ends.

2. Place in a bowl and top with applesauce, blackberries, and cinnamon. Serves 1.

Hemp Buckwheat

1 cup of hemp milk (see seed milk recipe)

⅓ cup buckwheat

2 tbsp. unsweetened applesauce

¼ cup raw walnuts

½ banana, chopped

½ tsp. hemp seeds

¼ tsp. cinnamon

¼ cup blueberries

Pinch ground Himalayan pink sea salt

Directions

1. Preheat oven to 350°F. Place walnuts on a baking sheet and roast for 8–10 minutes.

2. Bring hemp milk to a slight boil and whisk in buckwheat. Lower to simmer and cook for 10 minutes. Add salt just before cooking ends.

3. Place in a bowl or short glass, and top with applesauce, banana, walnuts, blueberries, cinnamon, and hemp seeds. Serves 1.

Walnut Oatmeal

1 cup walnut milk (see nut milk recipe)

⅓ cup gluten-free steel-cut oats

1 medjool date, chopped

2 tbsp. unsweetened applesauce

¼ cup fresh raspberries

½ fresh peach, diced

1 tsp. ground sesame seeds

¼ tsp. maca

¼ tsp. nutmeg

Pinch ground Himalayan pink sea salt (optional)

Directions

1. Bring walnut milk to a slight boil and whisk in oats, reduce to simmer and cook for 10 minutes. Add salt and chopped date just before cooking ends.

2. Place in a bowl and top with peaches, raspberries, maca, sesame, and nutmeg. Serves 1.

Goji Hemp Amaranth

1 cup hemp or almond milk (see seed or nut milk recipe)

1 tbsp. soaked (10 minutes in warm water)
   goji berries, drained and rinsed

½ banana

2 hemp bites, chopped (see resources)

1 chia bite, chopped (see resources)

1 apricot, chopped

1 medjool date, chopped

1 tsp. coconut nectar

1 tbsp. unsweetened coconut yogurt

½ tsp. cacao nibs

⅛ tsp. cloves

Directions

1. Bring plant milk and amaranth to a slight boil, reduce to simmer, and cook for 25 minutes.

2. Place in a bowl, and top with banana, coconut yogurt, goji berries, hemp bites, chia bite, apricot, date, cacao nibs, cloves, and coconut nectar. Serves 1.

Teff Porridge with Orange Macadamia Clove Cream

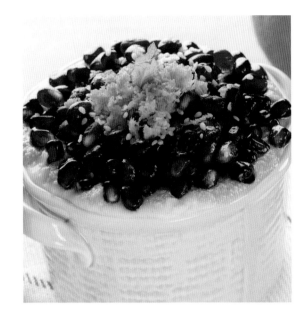

1 cup hemp milk (see
    seed milk recipe)

⅓ cup teff

⅛ tsp. ground Himalayan
    pink sea salt

⅓ cup soaked macadamia
    nuts, drained and rinsed

½ banana

Juice of ½ orange

1 tsp. orange zest

1 tsp. agave or coconut nectar

⅛ tsp. ground cloves

⅓ cup pomegranate seeds

½ tsp. sesame seeds

2 raw macadamia nuts

Directions

1. Bring hemp milk and teff to a slight boil, reduce to a low simmer,
    cover and cook for 15 minutes. Add salt just before cooking ends.

2. To make orange macadamia clove cream, place soaked
    macadamias, orange juice, banana, agave, and ½ the zest and
    cloves in a food processor and pulse until smooth.

3. Place teff porridge in a bowl or jar, top with orange macadamia
    clove cream, pomegranate seeds, sesame seeds, the rest of the
    orange zest and macadamia nuts. Serves 1.

Almond Oatmeal

1 cup almond milk (see
   nut milk recipe)
⅓ cup gluten-free steel-cut oats
¼ cup soaked (10 minutes in
   warm water) goji berries,
   drained and rinsed
Pinch ground Himalayan
   pink sea salt
1 tsp. chia seeds
1 tsp. coconut nectar
⅛ tsp. ginger
⅛ tsp. turmeric
⅛ tsp. cinnamon

Directions

1. Bring almond milk to a slight
    boil and whisk in oats, lower
    to simmer, and cook for 10
    minutes. Stir in goji berries and
    salt just before cooking ends.

2. Place in a bowl, top with chia,
    ginger, turmeric, cinnamon, and
    coconut nectar. Serves 1.

Rice Buckwheat

1 cup rice milk (see Tip
   on page 57)
⅓ cup buckwheat
¼ cup unsweetened applesauce
¼ cup raw or toasted, unsalted,
   chopped walnuts
¼ cup fresh blueberries
¼ tsp. cinnamon
Pinch ground Himalayan
   pink sea salt (optional)

Directions

1. Bring rice milk to a
    slight boil and whisk in
    buckwheat. Lower to
    simmer and cook for 10
    minutes. Add salt just
    before cooking ends.

2. Place in a bowl, and top with
    unsweetened applesauce,
    walnuts, blueberries, and
    cinnamon. Serves 1.

Cashew Amaranth

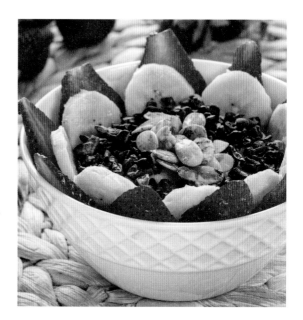

1 cup cashew milk (see
   nut milk recipe)

⅓ cup amaranth

⅓ cup sliced strawberries

½ banana sliced

1 tbsp. cacao nibs

1 tbsp. sprouted pumpkin seeds

1 tsp. agave (optional)

⅛ tsp. cinnamon

Directions

1. Bring cashew milk and amaranth to a slight boil, reduce to simmer, and cook for 25 minutes.

2. Transfer to a bowl, and top with strawberries, banana, cacao nibs, pumpkin seeds, agave, and cinnamon. Serves 1.

Hemp Oatmeal

1 cup hemp milk (see seed milk recipe)

⅓ cup gluten-free steel-cut oats

1 small chunk fresh ginger, peeled and finely grated

1 small chunk fresh turmeric, peeled and finely grated

½ cup fresh papaya, chopped

½ banana, diced

¼ cup blueberries

1 tsp. chia seeds

Pinch ground Himalayan pink salt

½ tsp. coconut nectar (optional)

Directions

1. Bring hemp milk to a slight boil, and whisk in oats, lower to simmer and cook for 10 minutes. Add salt, ginger, and turmeric just before cooking ends.

2. Place in a bowl and top with papaya, banana, and blueberries. Sprinkle on chia seeds and drizzle with coconut nectar (optional). Serves 1.

Oat Buckwheat

1 cup gluten-free oat milk (see Tip)

⅓ cup buckwheat

Pinch ground Himalayan pink sea salt (optional)

½ nectarine, sliced or chopped

2 tbsp. unsweetened applesauce

¼ cup blueberries

⅓ cup sliced strawberries

⅛ tsp. ground ginger

⅛ tsp. ground turmeric

⅛ tsp. ground cinnamon

Tip: To make oat milk, soak 1 cup of gluten-free oats in 4 cups of filtered water overnight. Place mixture in Vitamix or other high-powered blender along with 1–2 pitted medjool dates or 1 tbsp. coconut nectar, and blend on high for 1 minute. Pass through a nut strainer bag into a bowl. Any not immediately consumed can be stored refrigerated for 3–5 days.

Directions

1. Bring oat milk to a slight boil, and whisk in buckwheat, lower to simmer and cook for 10 minutes. Add salt just before cooking ends.

2. Place in a bowl and top with applesauce, nectarine, blueberries, strawberries, ginger, turmeric, and cinnamon. Serves 1.

Goji Hemp Buckwheat

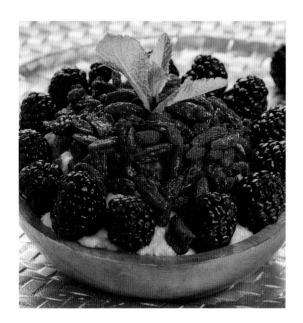

1 cup hemp milk (see
    seed milk recipe)

⅓ cup buckwheat

2 tbsp. soaked (10 minutes in
    warm water) goji berries,
    drained and rinsed

1 tsp. coconut nectar

¼ tsp. nutmeg

Pinch ground
    Himalayan pink sea salt

⅓ cup blackberries

Directions

1. Bring hemp milk to a slight boil. Whisk in buckwheat,
   reduce to simmer, and cook for 10 minutes. Add salt a
   couple of minutes before cooking ends.

2. Place in a bowl, top with blackberries and goji berries,
   drizzle on coconut nectar, and sprinkle with nutmeg.
   Serves 1.

Tip: Soaking goji berries for at least 10 minutes before consuming plumps them up and increases digestibility.

Creamy Walnut Goji Oatmeal

1 cup walnut milk (see nut milk recipe)

⅓ cup gluten-free steel-cut oats

⅓ cup soaked (10 minutes in warm water)
    goji berries, drained and rinsed

½ chopped banana

½ tsp. maca powder

½ tsp. coconut nectar or agave

⅛ tsp. coconut oil

⅛ tsp. ground ginger

⅛ tsp. ground turmeric

⅛ tsp. ground cinnamon

Pinch ground Himalayan pink sea salt

Directions

1. Bring walnut milk to a slight boil. Whisk in oats, lower to simmer, and cook for 10 minutes. Add goji berries, salt, and coconut oil a couple of minutes before cooking ends.

2. Transfer to a bowl, top with maca, banana, ginger, turmeric, cinnamon, and drizzle with coconut nectar or agave. Serves 1.

Goji Almond Buckwheat

1 cup almond milk (see nut milk recipe)

⅓ cup buckwheat

¼ cup soaked (10 minutes in warm water)
    goji berries plus 1 tsp. for topping

½ chopped banana

½ tsp. maca powder

1 tbsp. pistachios

¼ tsp. unsweetened coconut shreds

⅛ tsp. cardamom

½ tsp. coconut nectar

Directions

1. Bring almond milk to a slight boil. Whisk in buckwheat, lower to a simmer, and cook for 10 minutes. Add ¼ cup goji berries a couple of minutes before cooking ends.

2. Transfer to a bowl and top with maca powder, chopped banana, pistachios, 1 tsp. goji berries, coconut shreds, and cardamom and drizzle with coconut nectar. Serves 1.

Oatmeal with Strawberry Cream

1 cup cashew milk (see nut milk recipe)

⅓ cup gluten-free steel-cut oats

½ cup silken organic tofu

½ cup fresh strawberries or frozen strawberries

¼ cup soaked (10 minutes in warm water) goji berries,
    drained and rinsed

Zest and juice of ½ lemon

2 tsp. coconut nectar

½ tsp. coconut shreds

½ tsp. chia seeds

¼ tsp. ground Himalayan pink sea salt

1 strawberry halved

Directions

1. Bring cashew milk to a slight boil. Stir in oats, reduce to simmer,
    and cook for 10 minutes. Add salt and goji berries just before cooking
    ends.

2. To make strawberry cream, place silken tofu in a food processor
    with strawberries, agave nectar, lemon zest and juice, and pulse
    until smooth.

3. Place oatmeal in a bowl or short wide glass, and top with
    strawberry cream, coconut shreds, chia seeds, and 1 strawberry
    halved. Serves 1.

Hemp Walnut Amaranth

½ cup hemp milk (see seed milk recipe)

½ cup walnut milk (see nut milk recipe)

⅓ cup amaranth

½ chopped banana

¼ cup blueberries

2 tbsp. unsweetened applesauce

1 tsp. ground sesame seeds

½ tsp. coconut nectar or agave

⅛ tsp. ground nutmeg

Pinch ground Himalayan pink sea salt

Directions

1. Place plant milks and amaranth in a saucepan and bring to a boil. Lower to simmer and cook for 25 minutes, stirring occasionally. Add salt just before cooking ends.

2. Place in a bowl or short wide glass. Top with applesauce, ground sesame, banana, blueberries, nutmeg, and coconut nectar or agave. Serves 1.

Oatmeal with Hazelnut Strawberry Cream

1 cup hemp milk (see seed milk recipe)

⅓ cup gluten-free steel-cut oats

3 medjool dates, pitted

2 chia bites, chopped (see resources)

½ cup soaked hazelnuts

Juice of ½ lemon

½ cup strawberries

¼ tsp. ground Himalayan pink salt

1 tbsp. sprouted pumpkin seeds

1 strawberry, quartered

Directions

1. Bring hemp milk to a slight boil. Stir in oats, reduce to simmer, and cook for 10 minutes. Add salt and 1 date, chopped, just before cooking ends.

2. To make hazelnut strawberry cream in a food processor, pulse hazelnuts, strawberries, remaining dates, and lemon juice until almost smooth.

3. Place oatmeal in a bowl, top with hazelnut strawberry cream, chia bites, pumpkin seeds, and fresh strawberry. Serves 1.

Avocado Banana Buckwheat

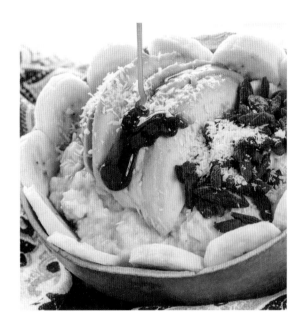

1 cup hemp milk (see
     seed milk recipe)

⅓ cup buckwheat

½ avocado, sliced

½ banana, sliced

¼ cup soaked (10 minutes in
     warm water) goji berries,
     drained and rinsed

Juice of ½ lime

1 tsp. coconut shreds

1 tsp. agave or coconut nectar

¼ tsp. ground Himalayan pink sea salt

Directions

1. Bring hemp milk to a slight boil. Stir in buckwheat,
   reduce to simmer, and cook for 10 minutes. Add salt and
   most of goji berries just before cooking ends.

2. Place in a bowl or short wide glass, and top with avocado,
   banana, coconut shreds, remaining goji berries, lime juice,
   and agave/coconut nectar. Serves 1.

Pumpkin and Walnut Oatmeal

1 cup hemp milk (see seed milk recipe)

⅓ cup gluten-free steel-cut oats

3 tbsp. unsweetened applesauce

½ banana chopped

1 tbsp. raw or roasted walnuts, chopped

1 tbsp. raw, sprouted pumpkin seeds

¼ tsp. ground Himalayan pink sea salt

⅛ tsp. nutmeg

1 tsp. coconut palm sugar or coconut nectar

Directions

1. Bring hemp milk to a slight boil, stir in oats, reduce to simmer, and cook for 10 minutes. Add salt just before cooking ends.

2. Place oatmeal in a bowl or short wide glass, and top with applesauce, banana, walnuts, pumpkin seeds, nutmeg, and coconut palm sugar/coconut nectar. Serves 1.

Cranberry Oatmeal

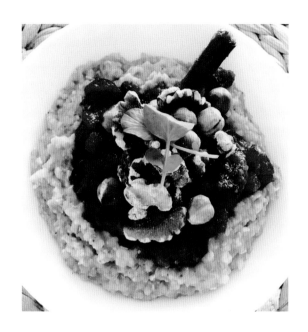

1 cup almond milk (see
　　nut milk recipe)

⅓ cup gluten-free steel-cut oats

3 tbsp. cranberry sauce (see
　　recipe on page 237)

¼ cup raw or toasted walnuts
　　and hazelnuts (see
　　roasting/toasting nuts)

¼ tsp. ground Himalayan pink salt

Directions

1. Bring almond milk to a slight boil, stir in oats, reduce to simmer, and cook for 10 minutes. Add salt just before cooking ends.

2. Transfer to a bowl or short wide glass, and top with cranberry sauce and nuts. Serves 1.

Teff Bowl

1 cup hemp milk (see seed milk recipe)

⅓ cup teff

½ banana sliced

¼ cup raspberries

¼ cup blueberries

1 tbsp. sprouted pumpkin seeds

1 tsp. hemp seeds

1 tsp. coconut nectar (optional)

⅛ tsp. ground Himalayan Pink sea salt

Directions

1. Bring hemp milk and teff to a slight boil, reduce to simmer, and cook for 15 minutes. Add salt just before cooking ends.

2. Top with sliced banana, raspberries, blueberries, pumpkin seeds, hemp seeds, and coconut nectar. Serves 1.

Coconut Oatmeal with Banana Matcha Cashew Cream

½ cup light coconut milk

½ cup water

⅓ cup gluten-free steel-cut oats

⅛ tsp. ground Himalayan pink salt

1 banana

1 tbsp. cashews, soaked overnight, drained and rinsed (see soaking nuts)

2 medjool dates, pitted

Juice of 1 lime

½ tsp. matcha green tea powder

⅓ cup fresh pomegranate seeds

½ tsp. raw sesame seeds

2 raw macadamia nuts

Directions

1. Bring coconut milk and water to a slight boil. Stir in oats, reduce to simmer, and cook for 10 minutes. Add salt just before cooking ends.

2. To make banana matcha cashew cream, place banana, cashews, dates, matcha, and lime juice in a food processor and pulse until smooth.

3. Place oatmeal in a bowl and top with banana matcha cashew cream, pomegranate seeds, sesame seeds, and macadamia nuts. Serves 1.

Buckwheat Bowl with Tahini Cream

1 cup hemp milk (see seed milk recipe)

⅓ cup buckwheat

⅛ tsp. ground Himalayan pink salt

Juice of 3 limes

4 medjool dates, pitted

1 tbsp. water

2 tbsp. sesame tahini

⅛ tsp. nutmeg

1 tbsp. soaked (10 minutes in warm water) goji berries

1 tsp. coconut shreds

½ banana, chopped

Tip: Left over tahini cream can be used in a workout recovery smoothie. See recipe on page 96.

Directions

1. Bring hemp milk to a slight boil. Stir in buckwheat, reduce to simmer, and cook for 10 minutes. Add salt just before cooking ends.

2. To make tahini cream, place lime juice, dates, water, tahini, and nutmeg in a food processor and pulse until smooth.

3. Transfer buckwheat into a bowl or wide short glass, and top with 2 tbsp. tahini cream, banana, goji berries, and coconut. Serves 1. Place leftover tahini cream in refrigerator. Consume within 3 days.

Apple Cashew Cream Amaranth

1 cup hemp milk (see seed milk recipe)

⅓ cup amaranth

3 tbsp. unsweetened applesauce

1 tbsp. raw cashew butter

¼ cup seedless black grapes, sliced

¼ cup raw, unsalted walnut pieces

¼ cup raspberries

½ tsp. coconut nectar or agave

Pinch ground Himalayan pink salt

⅛ tsp. nutmeg

Directions

1. Bring hemp milk and amaranth to a slight boil. Reduce to simmer, and cook for 25 minutes. Add a pinch of salt at the end of cooking.

2. To make apple cashew cream, blend or stir applesauce and cashew butter until well blended to a creamy texture.

3. Place cooked amaranth in a bowl or short wide glass. Top with apple cashew cream, walnuts, grapes, raspberries, nutmeg, and coconut nectar/agave. Serves 1. Delicious!

Plant Power Protein-Rich Granola

1 cup plant protein powder

1 cup chopped dried fruit (e.g. dates, figs, apricots)

1¼ cup chopped raw or toasted nuts

⅛ cup hemp seeds

⅛ cup chia seeds

4 cups gluten-free whole or rolled oats

1 tsp. maca

1 tsp. matcha green tea powder

½ cup shredded coconut

½ cup coconut nectar

½ cup agave

½ cup melted coconut oil

¼ cup melted cacao butter

¼ cup sprouted pumpkin seeds

¼ cup sprouted sunflower seeds

Directions

1. Preheat oven 325°F.

2. Place all dry ingredients in a food mixer and mix well.

3. In a separate bowl place coconut oil, cacao butter, agave and coconut nectar and stir until well mixed. Slowly add mixture to food mixer while it is running.

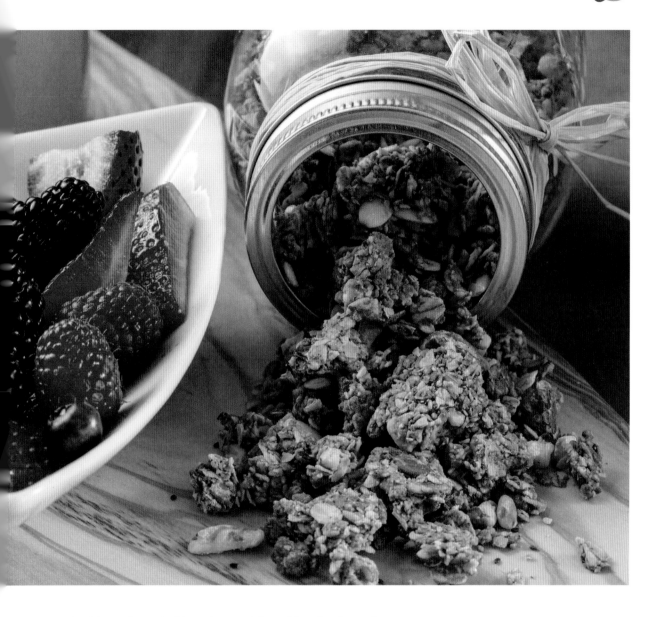

4. Line a large baking sheet with unbleached parchment paper, spread mixture out on baking sheet and flatten with the back of a spoon. Bake for 15 minutes.

5. When cooled breakup granola and store in a covered container refrigerated for up to 45 days.

Scrambled Tofu with Scallions and Shiitake Mushrooms

½ block extra-firm, tofu, crumbled

½ cup sliced shitake mushrooms

3 scallions, chopped

1 tsp. coconut amino acids

1 avocado, sliced

½ tsp. coconut oil

¼ tsp. smoked paprika

Salt and pepper to taste

Directions

1. Heat coconut oil in skillet over medium-high heat and add tofu, shiitakes, and scallions.

2. Sauté for 2 minutes and add amino acids.

3. Sauté for 1 more minute, sprinkle with smoked paprika, and top with avocado. Add salt and pepper to taste. Serve with coconut raisin quinoa. Serves 1.

Coconut Raisin Quinoa

2 cups vegetable broth

1 cup quinoa

½ cup raisins

1 tbsp. coconut shreds

¼ cup sprouted pumpkin seeds

2 tbsp. sliced almonds

Directions

1. Place vegetable stock and quinoa in a saucepan, bring to a boil, and simmer for 15 minutes, covered with a lid.

2. Fluff up and mix in raisins and coconut shreds, pumpkin seeds, and sliced almonds. Serves 2.

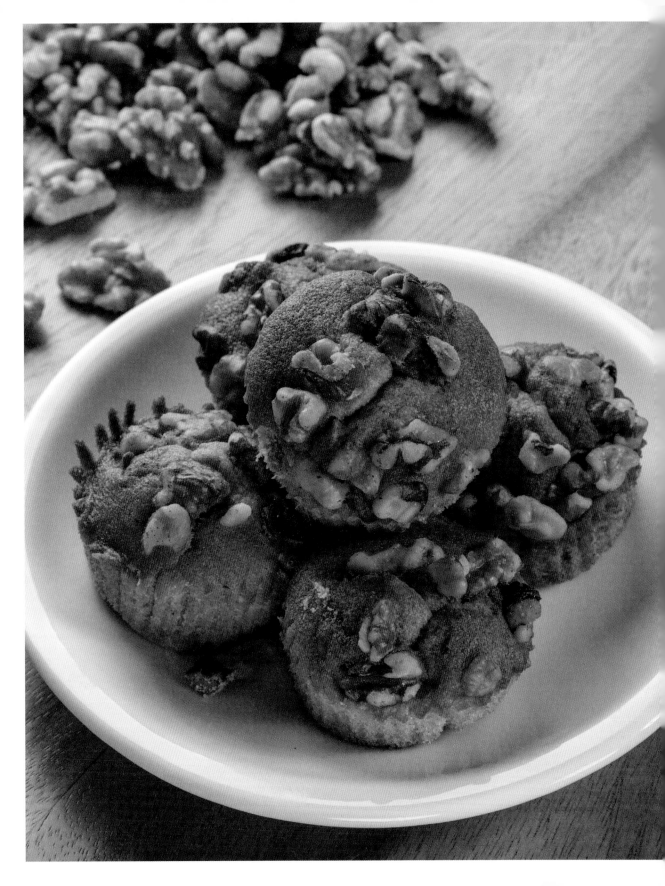

Muffins, Fruit Breads, and Pancakes

Muffins, fruit breads, and pancakes are also a great way to start your day, a good source of plant protein, high in fiber, and energy boosting. Make a whole batch, store them in the refrigerator, and enjoy as a quick breakfast on the go or energy snack between meals.

Banana Chocolate Chip Muffins

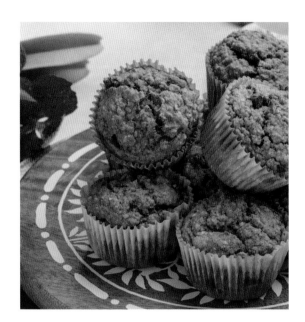

3 cups ground gluten-free
        oats or oat flour

2 tbsp. baking powder

2 tsp. vanilla bean powder

½ cup coconut sugar

1½ cups almond milk

4 tbsp. unsweetened applesauce

2 very ripe mashed bananas

½ cup vegan chocolate chips

Directions

1. Preheat oven 350°F. Place all dry ingredients in a large
    bowl and mix well.

2. In a separate bowl, place mashed bananas and applesauce
    and mix well.

3. Add plant milk to dry ingredients mixing well, add
    mashed banana and applesauce mixing well. Stir in
    chocolate chips and bake for 25 minutes. Makes 16
    muffins.

Carrot Raisin Walnut Muffins

1¼ cup gluten-free oat flour

¼ cup coconut flour

½ cup unsweetened applesauce

½ cup almond milk

½ cup raisins

1 cup grated carrot

½ cup chopped walnuts

⅓ cup coconut palm sugar

1 tbsp. baking powder

1 tsp. vanilla extract

1tsp. cinnamon

¼ tsp. Himalayan pink salt

Directions

1. Preheat oven 350°F. Mix flours in a large bowl, add baking powder, cinnamon, sugar and salt mixing well. Stir in milk, applesauce and vanilla extract being careful not to over-mix. Fold in carrots, raisins and walnuts. Transfer mixture to a muffin pan. Makes 12 muffins. Cook for 20–25 minutes.

Banana Macadamia Cream

Use to top fruit breads, muffins and pancakes.

½ cup soaked macadamia nuts, drained and rinsed well

Juice of 1 lime

4 soaked dates, pitted

1 tbsp. coconut milk

⅛ tsp. ginger

⅛ tsp. cinnamon

⅛ tsp. ground Himalayan pink sea salt

Directions

1. Place all ingredients in a food processor and pulse until smooth. Serves 2.

Banana Walnut Bread

1 cup ground gluten-free oats or oat flour

½ cup ground buckwheat or sweet sorghum flour

1 tbsp. baking powder

½ cup hemp milk

¼ cup gluten-free oat milk

⅓ cup ground golden flaxseed

1 ripe banana, mashed

2 tbsp. unsweetened applesauce

½ cup raw, unsalted, chopped walnuts

¼ cup coconut sugar

Pinch ground Himalayan pink sea salt

Directions

1. Preheat oven to 350°F.

2. In a large bowl combine oat flour, buckwheat flour, and baking powder, salt, and mix well.

3. In a small bowl combine mashed banana, applesauce, and coconut sugar, and mix well.

4. Add hemp milk and oat milk to dry ingredients and mix well.

5. Slowly add wet ingredients and mix well.

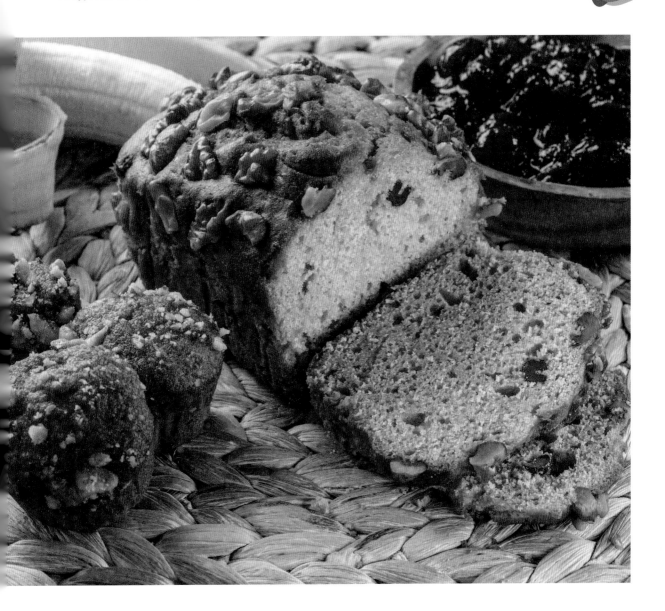

6. Stir in chopped walnuts, and transfer to a loaf tin or muffin pan.

7. If you have any extra chopped walnuts, add to the top with a little sprinkle of coconut sugar. Bake for 20–25 minutes for muffins, or 25–30 minutes for a loaf.

Blueberry Coconut Muffins

1½ cups gluten-free oat flour/
   ground whole oats

¾ cup sweet sorghum flour

¾ cup hemp milk

1 plain coconut yogurt

1¼ cups fresh blueberries

½ cup coconut sugar

⅓ cup unsweetened applesauce

1 tbsp. ground golden flaxseed

1 tbsp. baking powder

½ tsp. cinnamon

Directions

1. Preheat oven to 350°F.

2. Place all dry ingredients in a large bowl and mix well.

3. Place hemp milk, coconut yogurt, and unsweetened applesauce in another bowl, and mix well.

4. Add wet mixture to dry ingredients and mix well.

5. Stir in blueberries and spoon mixture into a nonstick muffin pan. Cook for 20–25 minutes. Makes 12 muffins

Suggested Topping: Pumpkin Seed Cream

½ cup soaked, raw pumpkin seeds, drained
   and rinsed (see soaking seeds)

½ banana

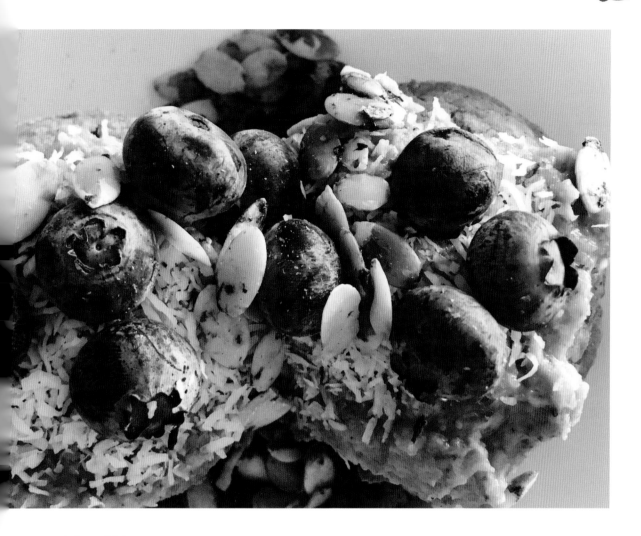

Juice of 1 lemon

3–4 medjool dates, pitted

Directions

1. Place all ingredients in a food processor and pulse until smooth.

2. Spread a little on each muffin, sprinkle with coconut shreds, blueberries, and sprouted pumpkin seeds.

Blueberry Buckwheat Pancakes

¾ cup ground buckwheat or buckwheat flour

1 tsp. lemon juice

1 tsp. baking powder

1 tsp. baking soda

¼ tsp. salt

½ tsp. vanilla extract

1 flax egg (1 tbsp. ground golden flaxseed plus 3 tbsp. water, mixed well)

1 tbsp. hemp oil

¾ cup hemp milk

2 tsp. coconut nectar

1 tsp. coconut oil

1 cup fresh blueberries

½ cup diced mango

Directions

1. Place all dry ingredients in a bowl and mix well.

2. In a separate bowl mix hemp milk with lemon juice and set aside for 5 minutes. Then add to dry ingredients mixing well. Add, hemp oil, flax egg, vanilla extract and coconut nectar mixing well.

3. Fold in half the blueberries.

4. Heat coconut oil on a griddle over medium high heat and add ¼ cup of mixture.

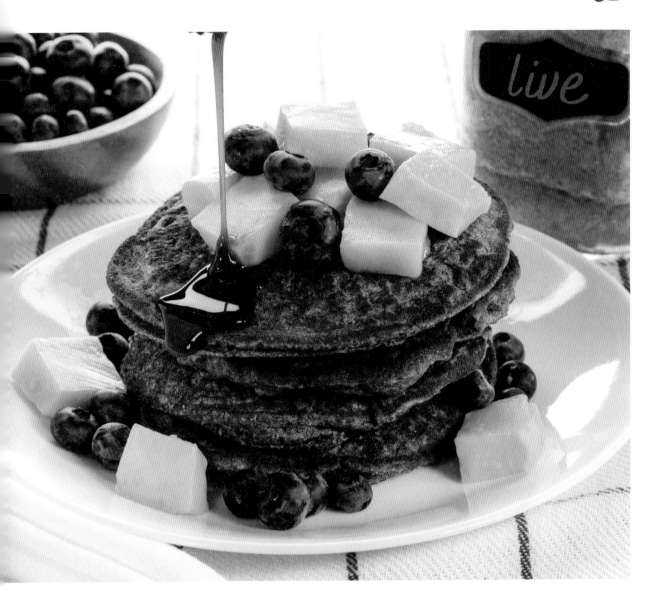

5. Cook until it begins to bubble a little in the center (about 3 minutes). Turn over pancake and cook for the same amount of time on the other side. Makes four pancakes.

6. After cooking, top with mango, remaining blueberries, and coconut nectar. Serves 2.

Strawberry Ginger Bread/Muffins

1¼ cups gluten-free ground
  oats or oat flour

¼ cup coconut flour

1 tbsp. baking powder

1 cup slightly pureed
  strawberries

1 tbsp. freshly grated ginger

⅓ cup coconut sugar

1 tsp. vanilla bean powder

2 tbsp. applesauce

¾ cup almond milk

Pinch ground Himalayan
  pink salt

Directions

1. Preheat oven to 350°F. Mix all dry ingredients together in bowl.

2. Blend milk, ginger, and coconut sugar, and mix into dry ingredients.

3. Stir in pureed strawberries and applesauce.

4. Place mixture in bread pan or muffin tin, top with gluten-free whole oats, and sprinkle a little coconut sugar on top.

5. Bake for 30 minutes for bread, and 20–25 for muffins.

Power Pancakes

1 cup buckwheat flour or ground buckwheat

1½ cups hemp milk or almond milk

½ cup light coconut milk

2 tbsp. hemp protein powder or 4 tbsp. ground hemp seeds

¼ cup ground golden flaxseeds

½ cup gluten-free oats

1 tbsp. baking powder

2 tbsp. unsweetened applesauce

¼ cup soaked (10 minutes in warm water) goji berries, drained and rinsed

¼ cup golden berries

1 tsp. cardamom

½ tsp. nutmeg

⅛ tsp. ground Himalayan pink salt

1 tbsp. agave

Directions

1. Place all dry ingredients in a large bowl and mix well.

2. Slowly add milk, applesauce, and agave, mixing well. Fold in goji berries and golden berries.

3. Cook on a griddle over medium-high heat with a little coconut oil, a few minutes each side. Top with Banana Macadamia Cream and fruit (see recipe on page 137). Serves 5 (1 pancake each).

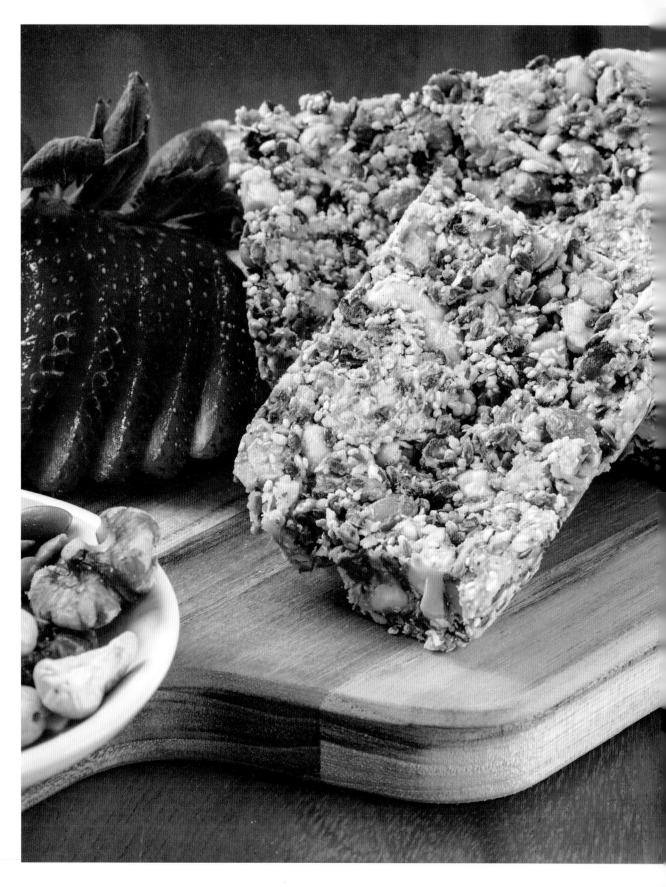

Live Bars

I decided to make these bars after searching the health food stores and being extremely disappointed with the majority of nutrition bars I found. Live Bars are loaded with superfoods, packing a nutrient-dense super-punch. They are incredibly delicious, and are great as a breakfast on-the-go, pre-workout snack, after-work-out snack, or between-meal snack. They are packed full of raw nuts and seeds, making them rich in protein and minerals. They also contain dried super fruits, which are packed with antioxidants, giving the immune system a boost!

Live bars need to be prepared the night before, and will stay fresh refrigerated for up to 45 days.

Live Power Bars

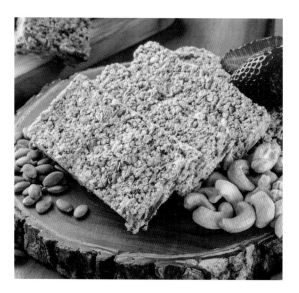

Power bars need to be prepared the day before.

1 cup of plant protein
    e.g. hemp powder

1½ cups chopped raw pecans

¼ cup chopped raw cashews

4 cups gluten-free oats

4 large medjool dates, chopped

2 large dried figs, chopped

¼ cup chia seeds

¼ cup sesame tahini

½ cup shredded coconut

1 tsp. cinnamon

¼ cup pumpkin seeds

¼ cup coconut oil

¼ cup cacao butter

4 tbsp. coconut nectar

¼ tsp. ground Himalayan
    pink sea salt

2 tsp. vanilla extract

Directions

1. Mix all dry ingredients first, then add dried fruit, tahini, coconut nectar, vanilla, coconut oil, and cacao butter.

2. Spread onto cookie sheet, making sure ingredients are flattened and leveled.

3. Store sheet in refrigerator overnight, and slice into bars the next day.

Super Nut Bars

1 cup raw, unsalted, roughly
   chopped macadamia nuts
½ cup raw, unsalted almond butter
1 cup raw, unsalted, roughly
   chopped Brazil nuts
4 tbsp. coconut nectar
½ cup cacao butter, melted
¼ cup pumpkin seeds
¼ cup cacao nibs
¼ cup hemp seeds

½ cup low-fat, shredded coconut
½ cup mulberries
¼ cup chia seeds
¼ cup sesame seeds
¼ cup flaxseeds
¼ cup sunflower seeds
1 tbsp. maca powder
1 tsp. vanilla extract
¼ tsp. ground Himalayan pink sea salt

Directions

1. Place all dry ingredients in a mixer and mix well.

2. Place almond butter, vanilla, and coconut nectar in a small bowl and mix well. Then add to dry ingredients while mixer is on.

3. Add melted cacao butter and transfer mixture to a cookie sheet. You can use unbleached parchment paper on cookie sheet if you like.

4. Make sure mixture is flattened out evenly with the back of a spoon.

5. Cover with unbleached parchment paper and place in refrigerator overnight. Slice into bars the next morning. The bars will keep for up to 45 days refrigerated.

Cacao Espresso Bars

1 cup raw, unsalted almonds, roughly chopped

½ cup raw, unsalted cashews, roughly chopped

½ cup raw, unsalted almond butter

5 tbsp. coconut nectar

⅓ cup pumpkin seeds

½ cup cacao butter, melted

⅓ cup soaked (10 minutes in warm water) goji berries, drained and rinsed

¼ cup chia seeds

2 tbsp. sesame seeds

½ cup low-fat, shredded coconut

¼ cup flaxseeds

⅓ cup raw, unsalted sunflower seeds

2 tbsp. cacao powder

¼ cup roasted espresso beans, in small pieces

1 tsp. cinnamon

1 tsp. chili powder

1 tsp. vanilla extract

¼ tsp. ground Himalayan pink sea salt

Directions

1. Place all dry ingredients in a mixer and mix well.

2. Place almond butter, vanilla, and coconut nectar in a small bowl and mix well. Then add to dry ingredients while mixer is on.

3. Add melted cocoa butter and transfer mixture onto a cookie sheet. You can use unbleached parchment paper on cookie sheet if you like.

4. Make sure mixture is flattened out evenly with the back of a spoon.

5. Cover with unbleached parchment paper and place in refrigerator overnight. Slice into bars the next morning. The bars will keep for up to 45 days refrigerated.

Walnut Crunch Bars

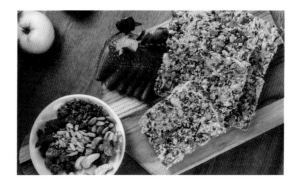

1 cup raw, unsalted walnuts, roughly chopped

1 cup raw, unsalted cashews, roughly chopped

½ cup raw, unsalted almond butter

4 tbsp. coconut nectar

½ cup cacao butter, melted

½ cup raw, unsalted pumpkin seeds

¼ cup hemp seeds

½ cup soaked (10 minutes in warm water) goji berries, drained and rinsed

¼ cup cacao nibs

¼ cup chia seeds

½ cup low-fat, shredded coconut

2 tbsp. sesame seeds

¼ cup flaxseeds

⅓ cup mulberries

1 tbsp. maca powder

1 tsp. vanilla extract

¼ tsp. ground Himalayan pink sea salt

Directions

1. Place all dry ingredients in a mixer and mix well.

2. Place almond butter, vanilla, and coconut nectar in a small bowl and mix well. Then add to dry ingredients while mixer is on.

3. Add melted cocoa butter and transfer mixture onto a cookie sheet. You can use unbleached parchment paper on cookie sheet if you like.

4. Make sure mixture is flattened out evenly with the back of a spoon. Cover with unbleached parchment paper and place in refrigerator overnight. Slice into bars the next morning. The bars will keep for up to 45 days refrigerated.

Super Green Bars

1 cup raw, unsalted almonds, roughly chopped

1 cup raw, unsalted cashews, roughly chopped

½ cup raw, unsalted almond butter

½ cup raw, unsalted pecans, roughly chopped

½ cup cacao butter, melted

½ cup raw, unsalted sunflower seeds

4 tbsp. coconut nectar

¼ cup hemp seeds

¼ cup cacao nibs

⅓ cup soaked (10 minutes in warm water) goji berries

½ cup mulberries

⅓ cup golden berries

¼ cup chia seeds

¼ cup low-fat, shredded coconut

1 tbsp. sesame seeds

1 tbsp. flaxseeds

1 tbsp. spirulina

1 tsp. chlorella

1 tbsp. camu camu powder

1 tsp. vanilla extract

¼ tsp. ground Himalayan pink sea salt

Directions

1. Place all dry ingredients in a mixer and mix well.

2. Place almond butter, vanilla, and coconut nectar in a small bowl and mix well. Then add to dry ingredients while mixer is on.

3. Add melted cacao butter and transfer mixture onto a cookie sheet. You can use unbleached parchment paper on cookie sheet if you like.

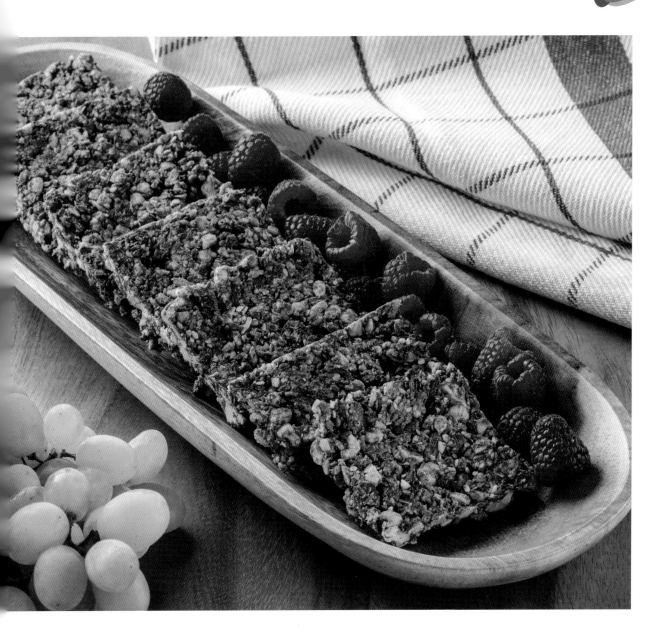

4. Make sure mixture is flattened out evenly with the back of a spoon. Cover with unbleached parchment paper and place in refrigerator overnight. Slice into bars the next morning. The bars will keep for up to 45 days refrigerated.

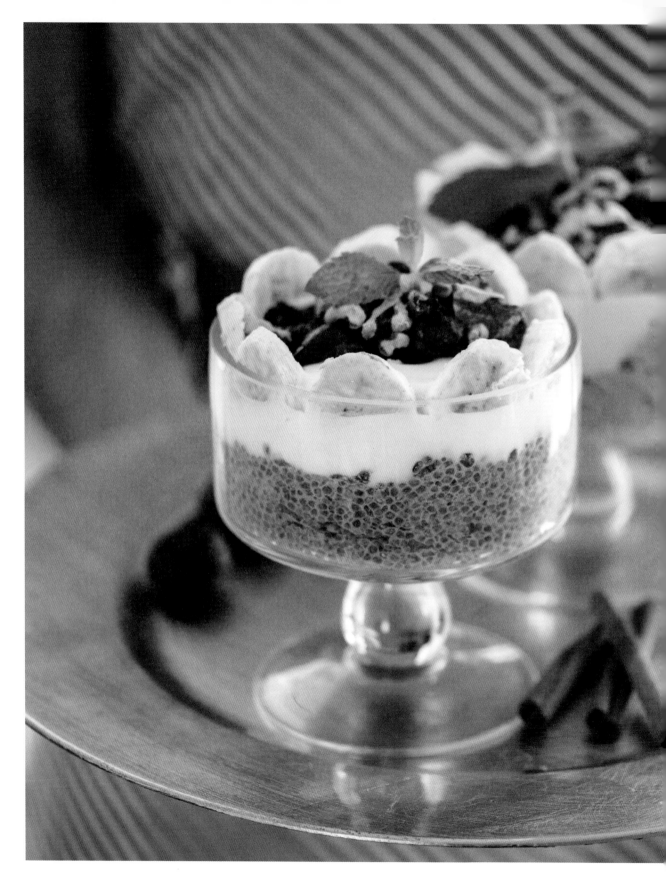

Chia Puddings

Chia puddings are a great way to start your day, or as an energy lifting snack, or dessert. Chia seeds date back to Mayan and Aztec cultures, and were believed to have supernatural powers. Not much has changed; chia seeds are still known as a superfood, providing long-lasting energy, and a high dietary-fiber source. Chia seeds contain omega-3 fatty acids, along with good amount of protein, magnesium, manganese, phosphorus, calcium, and iron. Check out my chia pudding recipes for a high-energy breakfast/snack/dessert! Chia puddings are best prepared the night before, covered, and refrigerated overnight.

White Chia Pudding with Cranberry Topping

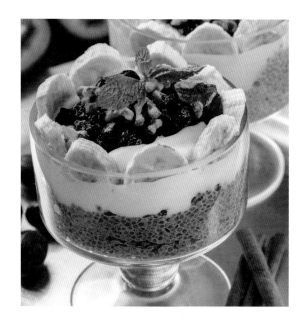

1 cup almond milk
   (see nut milk recipe)

¼ cup white chia seed

½ unsweetened coconut yogurt

½ banana sliced

⅓ cup cranberry sauce
   (see recipe on page 237)

¼ cup toasted/roasted walnuts

⅛ tsp. nutmeg (optional)

1 tsp. agave

½ tsp. vanilla extract

Sprig of fresh mint

Directions

1. Place almond milk, chia seed, agave, vanilla extract and nutmeg in a jar or measuring jug and hand whisk until it starts to thicken. Cover and refrigerate for 4 hours, or preferably overnight.

2. When ready, transfer to a dessert glass or leave in jar, and top with coconut yogurt, cranberry sauce, banana, walnuts and mint. Serves 1.

Green Chia Pudding

1 cup almond milk
  (see nut milk recipe)

¼ cup chia seeds

1 tsp. coconut nectar

½ tsp. vanilla extract

¼ tsp. spirulina

1 banana, sliced

¼ cup blueberries

Directions

1. Place almond milk in a bowl or measuring jug. Whisk in chia seeds, coconut nectar, vanilla extract, and spirulina.

2. Transfer to a glass or jar, cover, and refrigerate for at least 4 hours, preferably overnight. Before eating, top with sliced banana and blueberries. Serves 1.

Hemp Açaí Chia Pudding

1 cup hemp milk
  (see seed milk recipe)

¼ cup chia seeds

1 tsp. açaí powder

2 tsp. agave nectar

⅓ cup blueberries

Directions

1. Place hemp milk in a bowl or measuring jug. Whisk in chia, açaí, and agave until it is well mixed and starts to thicken.

2. Transfer to a glass or jar, cover, and refrigerate for at least 4 hours, preferably overnight. Before eating, top with blueberries. Serves 1.

Walnut Vanilla Chia Pudding

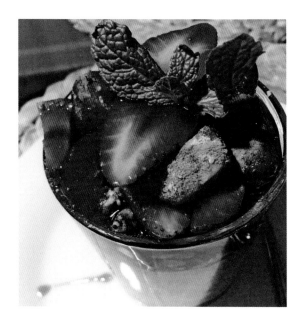

1 cup walnut milk
   (see nut milk recipe)

¼ cup chia seeds

1 tsp. coconut nectar or agave

½ tsp. vanilla extract

¼ tsp. cinnamon

⅓ cup sliced strawberries

½ tsp. maca

Directions

1. Place walnut milk in a bowl or measuring jug. Whisk in chia seeds, coconut nectar or agave, vanilla extract, and cinnamon.

2. Transfer to a glass or jar, cover, and refrigerate for at least 4 hours. Before eating, top with fresh, sliced strawberries and ¼ tsp. maca powder. Serves 1.

Cacao Chia Pudding with Macadamia Banana Coconut Cream

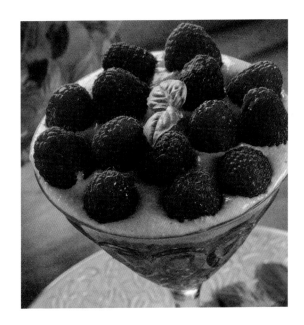

1 cup hemp milk
 (see seed milk recipe)

¼ cup chia seeds

1 tbsp. agave nectar

½ tsp. cacao powder

⅓ cup soaked, raw, unsalted
 macadamia nuts, drained and rinsed

1 banana

1 tbsp. coconut shreds

Pinch ground Himalayan pink sea salt

⅓ cup raspberries

1 sprig fresh mint or basil

Directions

1. Place hemp milk in a bowl or measuring jug. Whisk in chia, agave, and cacao powder until it is mixed well and starts to thicken.

2. Transfer to a jar, cover, and refrigerate for at least 4 hours, preferably overnight.

3. When chia pudding is ready, make macadamia banana coconut cream by placing macadamia nuts, banana, coconut, and salt in a food processor, and pulsing until well mixed and almost smooth.

4. Top chia pudding with macadamia banana coconut cream, raspberries, and sprig of mint/basil. Serves 1. Enjoy!

Maca Chia Pudding with Pomegranate

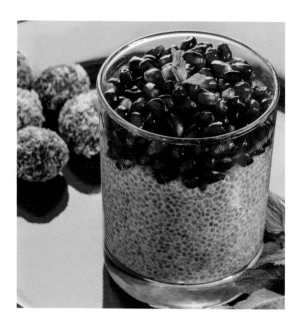

1 cup hemp or almond milk
    (see seed or nut milk recipe)

¼ cup chia seeds

½ tsp. maca

2 tsp. agave

½ cup fresh pomegranate seeds

Directions

1. Whisk up plant milk, chia seeds, maca, and agave until mixture starts to thicken.

2. Transfer to a glass or jar, cover, and refrigerate overnight.

3. In the morning, top with pomegranate seeds and enjoy! Serves 1.

Vanilla Chia Pudding with Kiwi

1 cup hemp or almond milk (see seed or nut milk recipe)

¼ cup chia seeds

2 tsp. agave

½ tsp. vanilla extract

2 tbsp. unsweetened applesauce

2 strawberries, sliced

1 kiwi, chopped

1 tbsp. toasted/roasted walnut pieces

⅛ tsp. cinnamon

Directions

1. Whisk plant milk, chia, agave, and vanilla until mixture starts to thicken.

2. Transfer to a glass or jar, cover, and refrigerate overnight.

3. In the morning, top with applesauce, strawberries, kiwi, walnuts, and cinnamon. Serves 1.

Matcha Green Tea Chia Pudding

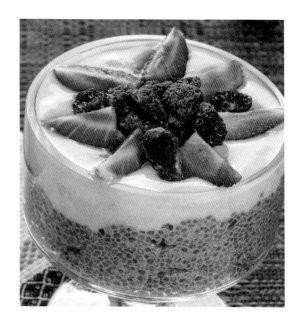

1 cup hemp milk
   (see seed milk recipe)

¼ cup chia seeds

½ tsp. matcha green tea powder

1 tsp. agave

1 banana

Juice of 1 lime

¼ cup sprouted sunflower seeds

⅓ cup strawberries

1 tbsp. golden berries

⅛ tsp. nutmeg

Directions

1. Whisk hemp milk, chia seeds, matcha, and agave until mixture starts to thicken.

2. Transfer to a jar, cover, and refrigerate overnight.

3. In the morning, place banana, lime, and sunflower seeds in a food processor, pulse until smooth, and use to top chia pudding. Add strawberries, golden berries, and nutmeg. Serves 1.

Vanilla Mulberry Chia Bowl

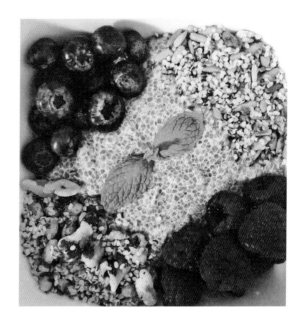

1 cup almond milk
   (see nut milk recipe)

¼ cup white chia seeds

1 tbsp. mulberries

1 tsp. agave

½ tsp. vanilla extract

¼ cup blueberries

¼ cup raspberries

1 tbsp. raw or toasted walnuts

1 tbsp. sprouted sunflower seeds

1 tbsp. hemp seeds

Sprig of fresh mint

Directions

1. Whisk almond milk, chia seeds, mulberries, agave, and vanilla extract until mixture starts to thicken.

2. Transfer to a jar or bowl, cover, and refrigerate overnight.

3. In the morning, top with the fruit, nuts, seeds, and mint.

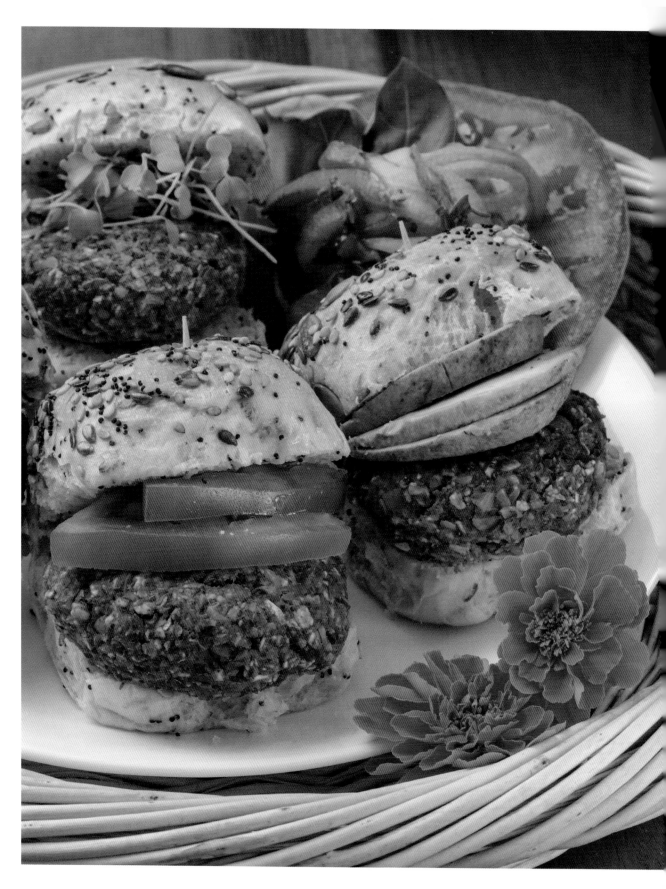

Main Dishes

CHAPTER

11

The following main dishes can be enjoyed for lunch or dinner, and are easy to prepare. They are plant-protein dense and complex-carbohydrate rich, making them high in fiber and low in fat. These dishes are not only delicious, but will also provide you with all the nutrients your body requires for long-lasting energy. Enjoy!

Chickpea (Garbanzo Bean) Curry

2 cups cooked chickpeas

2 onions chopped

4 large whole plum tomatoes

1 cup plain, unsweetened
    coconut yogurt

¼ cup sesame tahini

¼ tsp. turmeric

¼ tsp. ground Himalayan pink sea salt

1 tsp. chili powder

1 tsp. pressed ginger

1 tsp. garam masala powder

2 cloves garlic, minced

3 tbsp. poppy seeds

⅓ cup cilantro, chopped for garnish

Directions

1. To make coconut yogurt mixture, in a large bowl combine chickpeas, yogurt, turmeric, salt, ginger, garlic, and garam masala. Mix well and set aside.

2. To make tahini mixture, place tahini and poppy seeds in a food processor or blender and blend to a paste, adding water as necessary.

3. Heat a skillet over medium heat, and sauté onions.

4. Place thin cuts in whole tomatoes, add to onions, and cook for 10–15 minutes until soft enough to mash.

5. Add coconut yogurt mixture to tomatoes, and cook for 5 minutes. Add tahini mixture and cook for another 3–5 minutes.

6. Top with cilantro and serve. Serves 2.

Serve with brown basmati or jasmine rice.

Coriander Herb Roasted Potatoes

1 bag of small yellow
    potatoes, quartered

2 shallots, diced finely

1 clove garlic, minced

1 tbsp. olive oil

1 tsp. ground coriander

½ tsp. dried oregano

1 tsp. fresh thyme

¼ tsp. ground Himalayan
    pink sea salt

Directions

1. Preheat oven to 375°F. Place all ingredients in a large bowl and mix with a spoon to be certain potatoes are well coated with the other ingredients.

2. Spread evenly onto a baking sheet and roast for 30 minutes. Serve with ketchup (optional). Serves 4.

Brown Rice Salad

2 cups cooked, sprouted,
    short-grain brown rice

2 large tomatoes, chopped finely

4 green onions (scallions),
    chopped finely

½ red bell pepper, diced

½ yellow bell pepper, diced

1 cup fresh cilantro,
    finely chopped

¼ cup sprouted sunflower seeds

Zest from 1 lemon

1 large lemon, juiced

Pinch ground Himalayan
    pink sea salt

Pinch ground black pepper

Directions

1. Place cooked rice in a bowl, add vegetables, cilantro, zest, and sunflower seeds, and mix.

2. Add lemon juice, salt, and pepper to taste. Serves 2.

Lentil Loaf

2½ cup cooked sprouted lentils

2 purple carrots, diced

2 yellow carrots, diced

2 stalks celery, diced

1 cup bell peppers, diced
(mixture of red,
orange, and yellow)

2 cups chopped button
(white) mushrooms

½ cup chopped shitake
mushrooms

¼ cup quinoa flour

⅓ cup raw, unsalted,
chopped pecans

2 large cloves of garlic, minced

½ cup gluten-free oats

1 tbsp. fresh thyme

⅓ cup tomato paste

2 tbsp. nutritional yeast

½ onion, diced

2 tbsp. ground golden flaxseed

½ tsp. paprika

¼ tsp. ground Himalayan
pink sea salt

⅛ tsp. ground black pepper

1 tsp. Bragg or coconut
amino acids

1 tsp. coconut sugar

¼ cup ketchup

½ tsp. cayenne

1 cup gluten-free breadcrumbs

Directions

1. Preheat oven to 350°F.

2. Heat a large skillet, no need for oil, you can use a teaspoon of
vegetable broth if necessary. Sauté onions for 1 minute, then
add all other vegetables, garlic, thyme, salt, and pepper, and
sauté for 3 more minutes, and set aside.

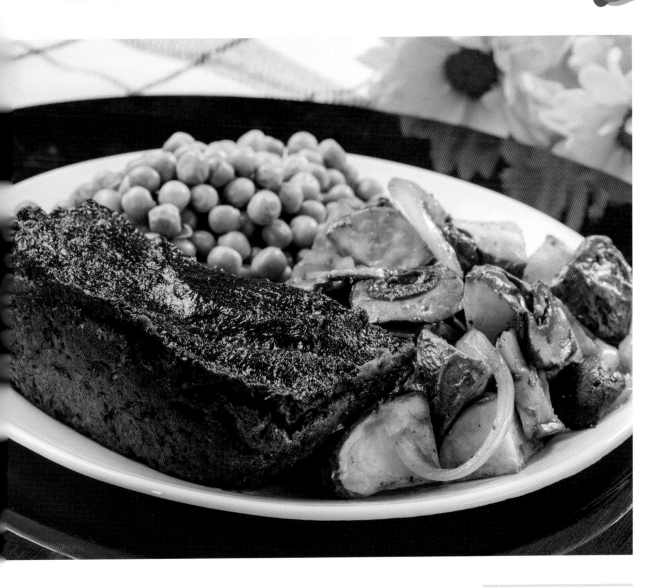

3. In a food processor, pulse lentils, vegetables, and all other ingredients, except ketchup.

4. Place in ceramic dish or loaf tin, cover, and cook for 30 minutes. Take out, top with ketchup, coconut sugar, and bake for an additional 10 minutes. Serves 8.

Tip: Use regular carrots if colors are not available (remember colored carrots are smaller so you will need less, so use 2 regular carrots instead of 4 colored carrots).

Red Kidney Bean Veggie Burgers

1½ cups cooked red kidney
    beans or 1 tin/carton
    drained and rinsed well

2 carrots, diced finely

2 stalks celery, diced finely

6 shiitake mushrooms,
    diced finely

½ sweet onion, diced finely

2 cloves garlic, minced

1 tbsp. ground golden flaxseed

1 tsp. coriander

1 tsp. cumin

½ tsp. onion powder

½ tsp. garlic powder

1 tsp. chilli powder

½ tsp. paprika

¼ cup gluten-free ground
    oats or oat flour

2 tbsp. ketchup

1 tsp. Bragg or coconut
    amino acids

¼ tsp. ground Himalayan
    pink sea salt

½ cup gluten-free breadcrumbs

Directions

1. Place kidney beans in a bowl and coarsely mash with a fork.

2. Heat a skillet over medium heat, and sauté onions for 2 minutes. Add carrots, celery, shiitake, garlic, salt, and 1 tsp. amino acids and sauté for 2 more minutes. Add coriander, chilli powder, paprika, cumin, onion powder, garlic powder, and sauté for 2 more minutes.

3. Add mixture from skillet to kidney beans and mix well.

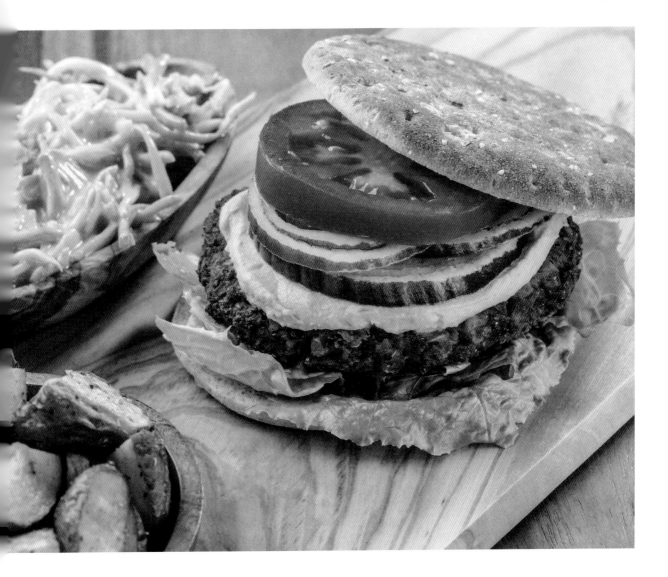

4. Add ketchup, flaxseed, breadcrumbs, and oat flour, while mixing well.

5. Make into 4 burgers and cook in a skillet with a little oil for 3 minutes on each side over medium heat. Or bake in the oven at 350°F for 10 minutes each side. Serve with Coriander Herb Roasted Potatoes (see recipe on page 167). Serves 4.

Garbanzo Beet Burgers

These veggie burgers can be eaten raw or cooked.
I prefer them raw topped on a salad.

3 cartons/tins of garbanzo beans,
  drained, rinsed and mashed

1 small sweet onion, finely chopped

1 carrot, grated

1 stalk celery, grated or finely
  chopped

¼ cup grated beet

½ cup finely chopped parsley

2 cloves garlic, minced

2 tbsp. raw, unsalted, ground
  cashews

½ cup quinoa flour

½ cup gluten-free ground whole oats

1 tbsp. ground golden
  flaxseed mixed with
  3 tbsp. filtered water
  (flax egg) or egg replacer

1 tbsp. ground cumin

1 tsp. Bragg liquid or
  coconut amino acids

1 tsp. vegan Worcestershire
  sauce

Pinch ground Himalayan
  pink sea salt (optional,
  amino acids and
  Worcestershire sauce
  contain enough sodium).

Directions

1. Pulse all ingredients in a food processor or mixer until
   mixed to a consistent texture. Form into burgers.

2. Enjoy raw, or sauté in a large skillet with very little oil
   (sesame or coconut) for 3–5 minutes each side. Or bake
   in the oven at 350°F for 10 minutes each side. Serves 8.

Black Bean Burgers

2 cartons/tins of black
beans, drained, rinsed
and roughly mashed

4 green onions (scallions),
chopped

½ cup gluten-free ground
whole oats

3 cloves of garlic, minced

1 red bell pepper, diced

½ cup organic corn

1 handful cilantro,
finely chopped

1 tbsp. cumin

1 tsp. tamari sauce

4 mini bello mushrooms,
chopped finely

Juice of 1 small lime

1 tsp. chili powder

1 tbsp. ground golden
flaxseed mixed with
3 tbsp. filtered water
(flax egg) or egg replacer

1 cup gluten-free whole oats

¼ tsp. ground Himalayan
pink sea salt

Directions

1. Pulse all ingredients in a food processor or mixer until
   mixed to a consistent texture. Form into burgers.

2. Enjoy raw, or sauté in a large skillet with very little oil
   (sesame or coconut) for 3–5 minutes each side. Or bake
   in the oven at 350°F for 10 minutes each side. Serves 4.

Curried Millet Balls

1 cup millet

2 cups vegetable broth

1 sweet/Vidalia onion,
    chopped finely

3–4 cloves of garlic,
    minced/pressed

1 tsp. vindaloo curry powder

½ tsp. paprika

2 tbsp. sweet white miso

3 tbsp. water

2 tbsp. tomato paste

2 tbsp. nutritional yeast

½ cup finely chopped cilantro

⅛ tsp. ground Himalayan
    pink sea salt

Directions

1. Preheat oven to 350°F.

2. Heat a large skillet over medium-high heat. Add sesame oil and toast ¼ cup of millet at a time to make sure it is toasted evenly or it will not cook evenly.

3. Place vegetable stock in a saucepan, add toasted millet, bring to a boil, reduce to simmer, cover, and cook for 25 minutes.

4. In a small bowl, mix miso paste and water well, and set aside

5. In a skillet, cook onions over medium heat for 5 minutes, adding a little vegetable stock if they become dry.

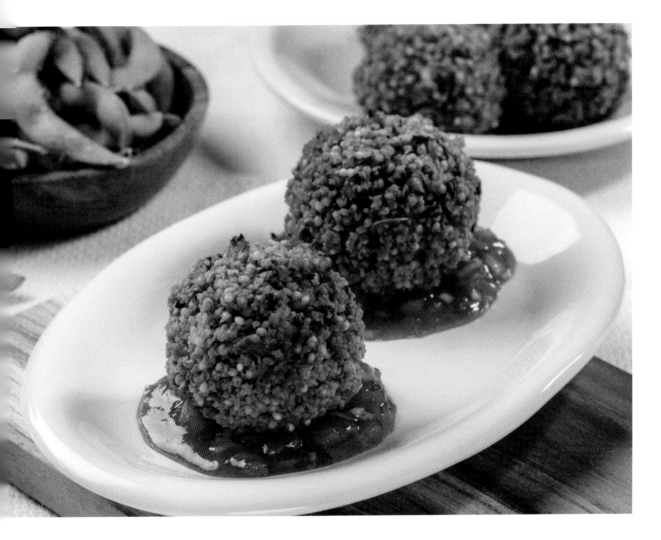

6. Add garlic, curry powder, paprika, and salt, and cook for 2 more minutes, adding a little vegetable stock if necessary.

7. Add miso mixture, tomato paste, and cilantro, and mix well.

8. Mold mixture into 12 small balls and place on a non-stick baking sheet, and cook for 20–25 minutes. Serve with apricot chutney or cranberry sauce (see recipes on page 236 and 237).

Baked Spaghetti Squash and Cannellini Bean Marinara

1 spaghetti squash

2 cups sun-dried tomato marinara (see recipe)

1 carton/tin cannellini beans, drained and rinsed

½ cup roughly chopped fresh basil and oregano

Pinch ground Himalayan pink sea salt

Directions

1. Preheat oven to 350°F. Cut spaghetti squash in half lengthwise, place both halves face down on baking sheet, and bake for 30 minutes.

2. Take out, turn over, and let cool enough to handle.

3. Add cannellini beans to marinara sauce and heat.

4. Scrape out spaghetti squash with a fork into a bowl, top with marinara, fresh basil, and salt.

Sun-dried Tomato Marinara

1 cup soaked sun-dried tomatoes

2 cloves garlic, minced

1 tin fire-roasted tomatoes

1 tbsp. balsamic vinegar

1 tbsp. hemp oil or olive oil

1 tsp. fresh thyme

1 tsp. dried oregano

Pinch ground Himalayan pink sea salt

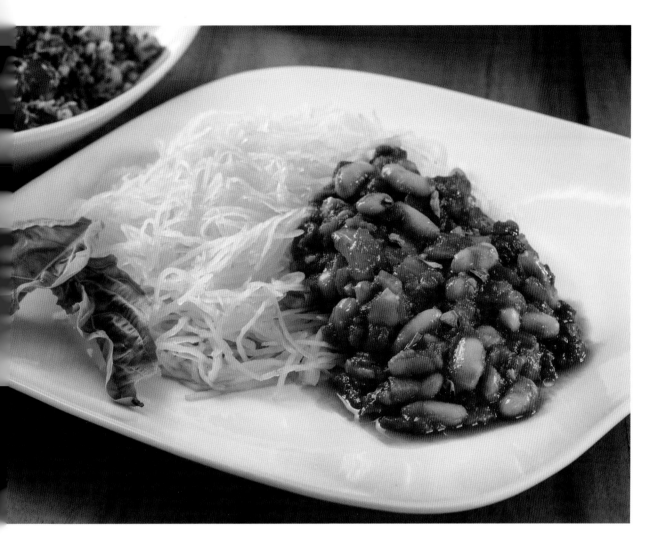

Directions

1. Place all ingredients in a food processor and pulse until almost smooth.

Sorghum Parsley Salad

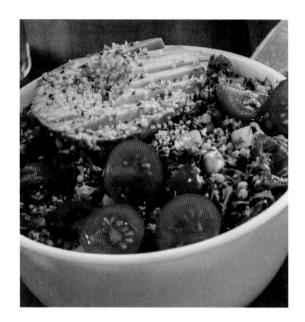

1 cup cooked sorghum

1 bunch parsley washed, dried
and chopped finely

1 bunch scallions chopped

1 cup cherry tomatoes quartered

1 avocado sliced

¼ tsp. pink Himalayan sea salt

¼ tsp. smoked paprika

zest and juice of 1 lemon

1 tsp. hemp seeds

Directions

1. Place sorghum, parsley, scallions, cherry tomatoes,
   salt and lemon zest and juice in a large bowl and mix
   well.

2. Top with avocado, smoked paprika and hemp seeds.
   Serves 2.

Creamy Cashew Mac and Cheese

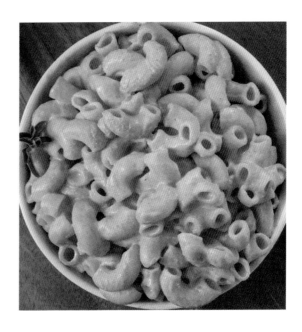

1 box ancient grain gluten-
   free pasta elbows

½ cup soaked, raw cashews,
   drained and rinsed

½ cup water

Juice of 1 lemon

1 red pepper, seeds removed
   and chopped

¼ cup nutritional yeast

2 tbsp. light coconut milk

1 tbsp. hemp oil or olive oil

1 tsp. garlic powder

1 tsp. onion powder

1 tsp. arrowroot powder

½ tsp. smoked paprika

¼ tsp. ground Himalayan
   pink sea salt

Cracked black pepper to taste

Directions

1. To make cashew cheese sauce, place all ingredients, except pasta elbows, into a blender or food processor, and blend until smooth.

2. Cook pasta according to directions on package.

3. In a separate saucepan, heat cashew cheese sauce gently over low heat until it starts to thicken.

4. Place pasta in bowl and top with creamy cashew cheese sauce. Serve Immediately! Serves 2–4.

Sweet Potato Beet Pizza

Pizza Crust – Sunflower and Sesame Seed

½ cup sprouted sunflower seeds

½ cup ground sesame seeds

½ cup quinoa flour

2 cloves minced garlic

1 tsp. fresh thyme or ½ tsp. dried

1 tbsp. sesame tahini

¼ cup olive or hemp oil

¼ tsp. ground Himalayan pink sea salt

Directions

1. Preheat oven to 375°F.

2. Place all ingredients in a food processor and pulse until a dough is formed.

3. Take out and flatten dough into a pizza pan. If you are concerned about sticking, you can dust it with a little quinoa flour.

4. Bake in oven for 15 minutes. Leave oven on.

Pizza Topping

1 cup sun-dried tomato marinara
    sauce (see recipe on page 233)

½ cup grated sweet potato

½ cup grated beets

½ cup sliced red pepper

⅓ cup sliced sweet onion

1 large sliced tomato

½ cup finely chopped parsley

½ cup roughly chopped basil

¼ cup cashew parmesan (see
    recipe on page 241)

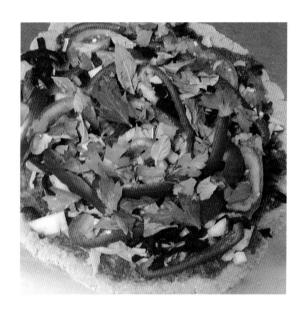

Directions

1. Top crust with marinara sauce, sliced onion, and red
   pepper. Top with grated carrot, beets and sliced tomato,
   and sprinkle with cashew parmesan.

1. Bake for 25 minutes.

2. Take out of oven and top with parsley and basil, and
   serve. Serves 2.

Watercress Chopped Salad, Roasted Sweet Potatoes, and Brown Basmati Ginger Coconut Rice

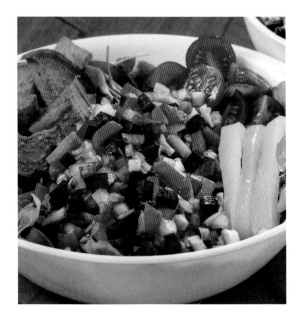

2 cups watercress

1 cup Roasted Sweet Potatoes (see recipe on page 208)

1 cup chopped salad (mix of beets, carrots, celery, cucumber and onion)

½ cup halved cherry tomatoes

⅓ cup sliced yellow peppers

1 cup Brown Basmati Ginger Coconut Rice (see recipe on page 221)

½ cup English peas

¼ cup pistachios

Directions

1. Place watercress in a salad bowl, and top with sweet potatoes, tomatoes, chopped salad and yellow peppers. Serve with brown basmati ginger coconut rice topped with English peas and pistachios. Serves 1–2

◀ Suggested salad dressing: Lemon Herb Garlic Vinaigrette (see recipe page 250)

Smokey Coconut Red Rice Salad

1 cup cooked red rice

2 carrots peeled

2 stalks celery

1 radish

⅓ cucumber

⅓ bell red pepper

¼ sweet/Vidalia onion

¼ cup shelled pistachios

1 tbsp. coconut shreds

2 tbsp. ground sesame seeds

2 tomatoes, quartered

Zest of 1 lemon

1 lemon, juiced

1 tbsp. raisins

½ tsp. smoked paprika

2 tsp. olive oil

⅛ tsp. ground Himalayan
    pink sea salt

⅛ tsp. ground black pepper

Directions

1. Chop carrots, celery, radish, cucumber, bell pepper, and onion in a chopper.

2. Place 1 cup cooked red rice in a large bowl. Add pistachios, sesame seeds, coconut shreds, raisins, lemon zest, and smoked paprika, and mix well.

3. Stir in chopped vegetables, lemon juice, olive oil, salt, and pepper, mixing well. Serves 2.

Mushroom Broccolini Quinoa and Pinto Marinara served with Creamy Avocado Kale

2 cups vegetable stock

1 cup quinoa

1 cup sliced baby portobello
   mushrooms

1 onion, sliced

2 cloves garlic, minced

1 bunch broccolini washed,
   just the ends of the
   stalks trimmed

1 bunch dinosaur kale, washed
   and shredded finely

2 cups marinara sauce (see
   recipe on page 233)

1 tin/can pinto beans,
   drained and rinsed

1 avocado

1 clove garlic

1 lime, juiced

1 tsp. balsamic vinegar

¼ tsp. ground Himalayan
   pink sea salt

1 tsp. hemp oil

½ cup water

⅓ cup frozen mango

2 tsp. coconut amino acids

1 small date or ½ medjool date

Directions

1. Place vegetable stock and quinoa in a saucepan and
    bring to a slight boil, cover, and simmer for 15 minutes.

2. Heat a large skillet over medium heat and sauté onions
    for 1 minute. Add 1 tsp. coconut amino acids and sauté
    until onions begin to caramelize. Remove onions and set
    aside.

3. In the same skillet sauté mushrooms and broccolini in balsamic vinegar for 1 minute. Add garlic and salt, and sauté 2 more minutes. Set aside.

4. Heat marinara and pinto beans together. Place pinto marinara in a dish and cover.

5. Place cooked quinoa in a large serving dish, top with cooked broccolini, mushrooms, garlic, and, lastly, caramelized onions. Cover dish, and set aside.

6. To make creamy avocado dressing, place avocado, lime juice, hemp oil, water, frozen mango, 1 tsp. coconut amino acids, and date in a blender until smooth.

7. First serve kale topped with creamy avocado dressing, followed by mushroom, broccolini quinoa and pinto marinara. Serves 2.

Parsley and Mint Salad

1 bunch flat-leaf parsley, finely chopped

½ cup roughly torn mint leaves

1 large tomato, finely chopped, seeds removed

3 scallions, finely chopped

½ tsp. chopped roasted garlic

½ lemon, juiced

1 tsp. olive oil

Pinch ground Himalayan pink sea salt

Pinch cracked black pepper

Directions

1. In a bowl mix all ingredients and enjoy! Serves 1–2.

Black Bean Quinoa Burgers

2½ cups of cooked black
beans or 2 tins/cartons
drained and rinsed

1½ cups cooked quinoa

2 cloves garlic minced

½ sweet onion finely chopped

1 carrot finely chopped

1 stalk celery finely chopped

⅓ cup soaked walnuts

1 tsp. cumin

1 tsp. paprika

¼ tsp. salt

1 tbsp. vegan barbecue sauce

1 tsp. coconut amino acids

Directions

1. Preheat oven to 350°F.

2. Place black beans in a food processor, and pulse until roughly chopped.

3. Heat a skillet over medium and sauté onions for 2 minutes. Add carrots, celery and garlic and cook for 2 more minutes, adding coconut amino acids to prevent from drying out. Remove from heat and stir in salt, cumin, and paprika.

4. Add cooked vegetables to the beans in the food processor, along with walnuts, quinoa, and barbecue sauce. Pulse until ingredients are mixed well.

5. Using a non-stick baking sheet or lining one with unbleached parchment paper, mold mixture into 6 burgers, and place on sheet. Cook for 10 minutes each side.

Roasted Potatoes, Beets, and Carrots

10 small yellow potatoes, quartered

3 carrots, peeled and sliced into large pieces

1 beet, peeled and cut into large chunks

3 cloves garlic, pressed or minced

½ tsp. dried sage

½ tsp. dried rosemary

½ tsp. dried thyme

1 tbsp. olive oil

½ tsp. ground Himalayan pink sea salt

Directions

1. Preheat oven to 400°F.

2. In a large bowl, mix all ingredients until vegetables are well coated.

3. Spread out mixture on a baking sheet and roast for 25–30 minutes. Serve with Watercress Tendril and Lentil Salad (see recipe on page 220). Serves 2–3.

Spinach Salad

4 cups fresh baby spinach

1 cup grape or cherry tomatoes, halved

1 cup sliced yellow bell pepper

½ cup sliced button (white) mushrooms

⅓ sweet onion, sliced

⅓ cup diced cucumber

½ cup shredded or grated carrots

3 tbsp. aged balsamic vinegar

2 tbsp. extra virgin olive oil

1 tbsp. nutritional yeast

Ground Himalayan pink sea salt and
 ground black pepper to taste

Directions

1. Place all vegetables in a salad bowl and sprinkle nutritional yeast on top.

2. Toss with olive oil, balsamic vinegar, salt, and pepper. Serve with coconut raisin quinoa. Serves 2.

Coconut Raisin Quinoa

2 cups vegetable broth

1 cup quinoa

½ cup raisins

1 tbsp. coconut shreds

¼ cup sprouted pumpkin seeds

2 tbsp. sliced almonds

Salt to taste

Directions

1. Place vegetable stock and quinoa in a saucepan, bring to a boil, and simmer for 15 minutes covered with a lid.

2. Fluff up. Add raisins, coconut, almonds, and pumpkin seeds. Serve over spinach salad. Serves 2–4.

Pineapple Cashew Stir Fry and Wild Rice

1 cup mixed wild rice

1¾ cups vegetable stock

⅓ cup raw, unsalted cashews

2 cloves of garlic minced

½ red bell pepper, sliced

5 green onions (scallions), chopped

½ cup shitake mushrooms, sliced

½ cup fresh pineapple chunks

½ cup sliced carrots

½ cup sliced celery

1 tsp. sesame oil

2 tbsp. vegetable stock

1 tsp. tamari sauce

Ground Himalayan pink sea salt to taste

Directions

1. Place wild rice and vegetable stock in a saucepan and bring to a boil. Reduce to simmer, cover, and cook for 45 minutes. Then uncover and set aside.

2. Heat dry large skillet on medium high, and toast cashews for a couple minutes until golden brown. Remove cashews and set aside.

3. In the same skillet, heat sesame oil on medium high. Add garlic to skillet along with all vegetables and pineapple, and sauté for 3 minutes. Add 2 tbsp. vegetable stock, tamari sauce, and cashews, turn off heat. Serve with wild rice. Serves 2.

Red Rice Sprouted Lentil Burgers

1½ cups cooked sprouted lentils

1 cup cooked red rice

½ cup cooked sweet potato

1 cup gluten-free ground rolled oats or quick-cooking oats

½ cup soaked raw unsalted walnuts, drained and rinsed

½ sweet onion, chopped

¼ cup ground golden flaxseed

¼ cup ketchup or tomato paste

2 cloves garlic, minced

1 tbsp. whole-grain Dijon mustard

1 tsp. smoked paprika

1 tsp. chilli powder

¼ tsp. ground Himalayan pink sea salt

¼ tsp. ground black pepper

Directions

1. Preheat oven to 375°F.

2. Place onions, garlic, sweet potato, and walnuts in a food processor and pulse until mixed.

3. Add rice and lentils, and pulse until mixed well.

4. Transfer mixture to a bowl and add paprika, chilli powder flax, ketchup, Dijon mustard, oats, salt, and pepper, and mix well.

5. Make into 6 burgers. Cover a baking sheet with unbleached parchment paper, and place burgers on sheet. Cook 10 minutes each side.

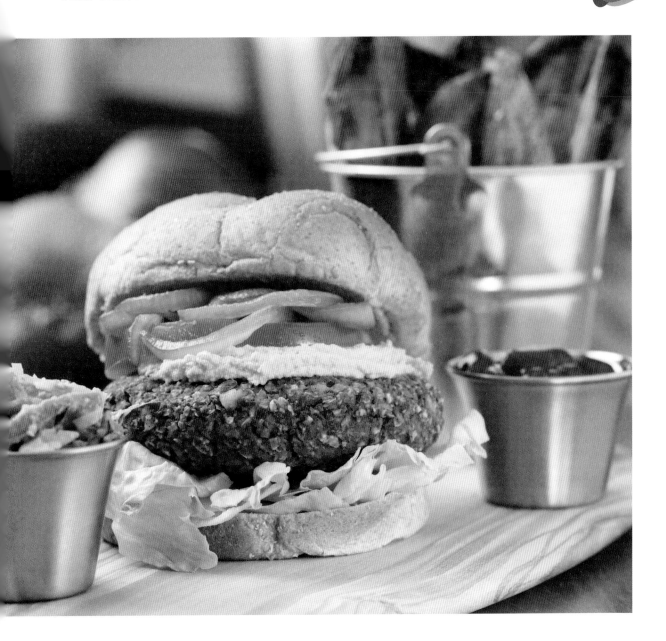

6. Serve on a whole-grain gluten-free bun and top with
   cashew cheese (see recipe on page 248), fresh tomato, red
   onion, and avocado.

Millet Veggie Cakes

2 cups cooked millet

½ onion, chopped

2 cloves garlic

2 carrots, roughly chopped

2 stalks celery, roughly chopped

2 cups parsley, stalks removed

¼ cup raw or roasted cashews

1 tbsp. ground sesame seeds

1 tbsp. egg replacer or ground
golden flaxseed (mix
either one with 3 tbsp.
water just before using)

½ lemon, juiced

½ cup quinoa flour or
millet flour

1 tsp. coconut amino acids

1 tsp. vegan Worcestershire
sauce

1 tsp. smoked paprika

1 tsp. cumin

¼ tsp. ground Himalayan
pink salt

¼ tsp. cracked black pepper

½ tsp. of chilli powder or
¼ tsp. cayenne

Directions

1. Preheat oven to 375°F.

2. Pulse parsley, garlic, onions, carrots, and celery in a food
processor until chopped finely and mixed well.

3. Add cashews, lemon juice, salt, and pepper, and pulse
until mixed well.

4. Add millet and pulse until mixed well.

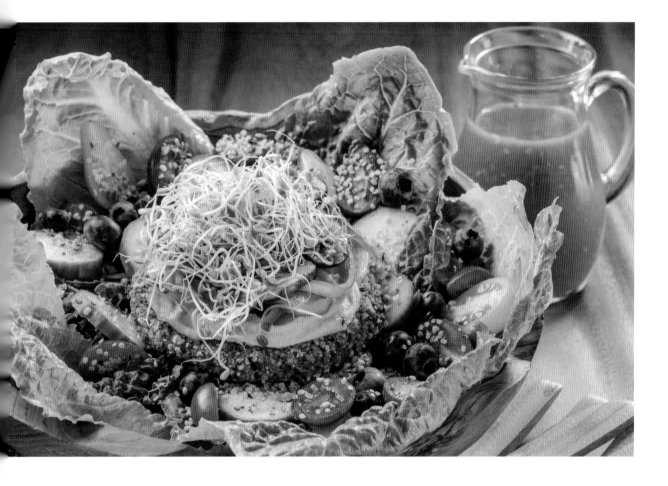

5. Transfer to a large bowl, and add paprika, cayenne, cumin, coconut amino acids, and Worcestershire sauce, and mix well.

6. Add quinoa flour and egg replacer/flax mixed with water.

7. Line a baking sheet with unbleached parchment paper.

8. Form mixture into 6 good-sized patties, and bake for 10 minutes each side.

9. Top with cashew cheese (see recipe on page 248) and caramelized onions.

Roasted Eggplant and Sweet Potatoes with Sprouted Lentil Ragu and Coconut Cheese Sauce

1 large eggplant washed and
    cut into 1 inch chunks

2 sweet potatoes washed and
    cut into 1 inch chunks

2 tbsp. fresh ground rosemary,
    sage and thyme

3–4 cloves garlic minced

½ tsp. pink Himalayan sea salt

2 tbsp. olive oil

Directions

1. Preheat oven to 375°F. Place all ingredients in a large bowl and mix well.

2. Spread mixture out on a large baking sheet and cook for 30–35 minutes.

Sprouted Lentil Ragu

1 cup sprouted green lentils

3 cups vegetable stock

½ sweet/Vidalia onion chopped

1 carton/can fire roasted
    tomatoes

¼ cup fresh oregano

¼ tsp. onion powder

¼ tsp. garlic powder

2 bay leaves

¼ tsp. pink Himalayan sea salt

1 tbsp. olive oil

2 cloves garlic minced

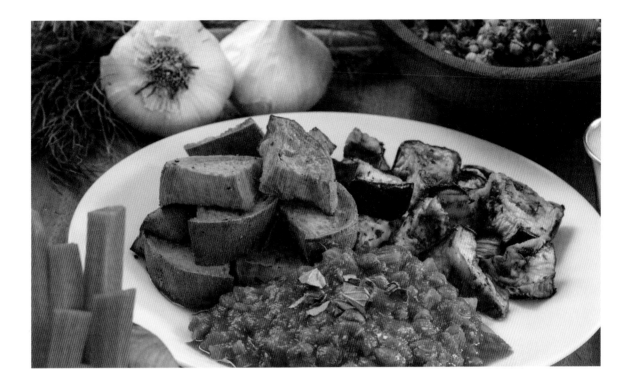

Directions

1. Place lentils, vegetable stock, 1 bay leaf, onion powder and garlic powder in a saucepan and bring to a boil. Lower to simmer and cook for 30 minutes.

2. Heat a skillet over medium heat and add oil and onion. Cook for 2 minutes. Add garlic and cook for 2 minutes. Add bay leaf and tomatoes and cook for 5 minutes. Add lentils and simmer for 5 more minutes.

3. Top with fresh oregano. Serves 2.

Coconut Cheese Sauce (see recipe on page 253)

Stuffed Acorn Squash

1 acorn squash cut in
    half lengthwise, seeds
    scooped out

1 cup brown, short-grain rice

2 cups vegetable stock
    plus 2 tsp. extra

2 carrots, peeled and finely diced

2 stalks celery, finely diced

½ sweet/Vidalia onion,
    finely diced

1 clove garlic, minced

¼ cup raisins

¼ cup pine nuts

1 tbsp. unsweetened
    coconut shreds

1 tsp. cumin

½ tsp. oregano

½ tsp. ground sage

2 tsp. olive oil

½ tsp. ground Himalayan
    pink sea salt

Directions

1. Preheat oven to 375°F.

2. Place rice in a saucepan with 2 cups vegetable stock, bring
    to a boil, and simmer for 45 minutes.

3. Coat inside of acorn squash with 1 tsp. of olive oil and ¼
    tsp. sea salt.

4. Place face up on baking sheet, place in oven, and cook for
    30–45 minutes.

5. Heat 1 tsp. olive oil in a large skillet over medium heat,
    add onions and sauté for 1 minute.

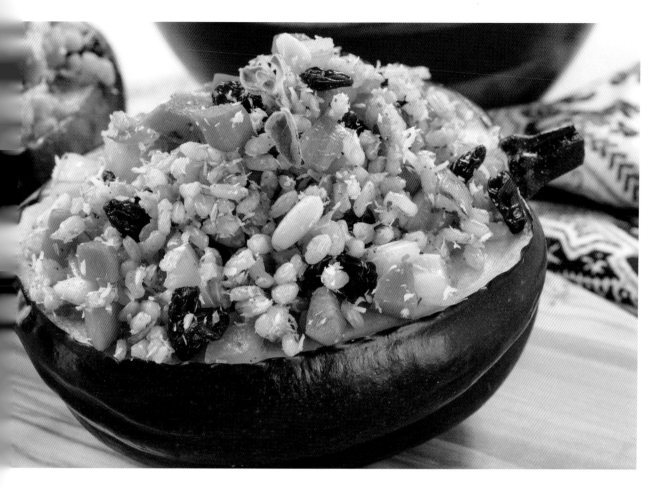

6. Add celery, carrot, garlic, oregano, sage, and salt, and cook for 3 more minutes. If it seems too dry, add 2 tsp. vegetable stock. Set aside.

7. Once rice is cooked, add to cooked vegetables, along with raisins, coconut, pine nuts, and cumin, and mix well.

8. Once squash is cooked, take out of oven, fill with rice mixture, and serve.

9. Serve with Parsley and Mint Salad (see recipe on page 185). Serves 2.

Baked Portobello Mushrooms

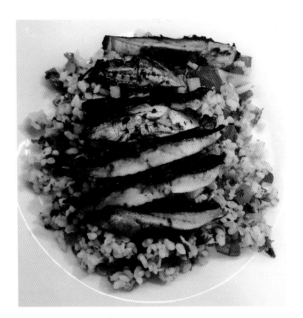

2 large portobello mushrooms

3 cloves garlic, minced

1 tbsp. grated fresh ginger

2 tbsp. coconut amino acids

2 tsp. vegan Worcestershire sauce

1 tbsp. tamari sauce

2 tbsp. balsamic vinegar

1 tsp. coconut nectar

Pinch ground black pepper

Directions

1. Place mushrooms stem side up, side by side, in a dish.

2. Mix all remaining ingredients into a marinade and pour over mushrooms, cover, and allow to marinate for at least 1 hour.

3. Preheat oven to 375°F.

4. Bake in oven for 15 minutes.

5. Take out, turn over mushrooms, top with any remaining marinade, and cook an additional 15 minutes.

6. Take out and allow to cool for 5 minutes before cutting into slices. Serve on top of Brown Rice Salad (see recipe on page 167). Serves 2.

Quinoa Kidney Bean Burgers

1½ cups cooked kidney beans or 1 carton/tin, drained and rinsed

⅔ cup cooked quinoa

1 cup grated carrot

⅓ cup minced onion

1 garlic clove, minced

⅓ cup quinoa flour

⅓ cup ground sprouted pumpkin seeds

2 tbsp. vegetable stock

1 tbsp. apple cider vinegar

1 tbsp. egg replacer or ground flaxseed mixed with 2 tbsp. water

Juice of ½ lime

1½ tsp. cumin

1 tsp. smoked paprika

1 tsp. pumpkin seed oil or olive oil

1 tsp. coconut or Bragg amino acids

Directions

1. Place kidney beans in a food processor and pulse until coarse.

2. Add all other ingredients, and pulse until mixed well.

3. Form into burgers. Makes 6 small burgers.

4. Heat griddle with a little olive or sesame oil on medium heat, and cook burgers 3 minutes each side, or cook in oven at 350°F for 10 minutes each side. Serves 4–6.

Red Quinoa Stir Fry with Baked Sweet Potato Hazelnut Fries

½ cup red quinoa

2 cups vegetable stock plus 2 tsp. extra

1 bunch curly parsley, washed and chopped finely

3 carrots, peeled and diced finely

3 stalks celery, diced finely

1 clove elephant garlic, minced

¼ cup raisins

1 tbsp. unsweetened coconut shreds

½ tsp. oregano

½ tsp. ground sage

1 tsp. cumin

1 tsp. olive oil

¼ tsp. ground Himalayan pink sea salt

¼ tsp. cracked black pepper

1 tbsp. apple cider vinegar

1 tbsp. ketchup

Directions

1. Prepare sweet potato fries (see recipe on page 201).

2. Bring vegetable stock and quinoa to a slight oil, reduce to simmer and cook for 15–20 minutes.

3. Place carrots, celery, and garlic in a bowl. Add 1 tsp. olive oil, sage, oregano, salt, and pepper and mix well.

4. Heat a skillet on medium. Add onion and sauté for 1 minute.

5. Add mixed vegetable ingredients from bowl and sauté for 3 more minutes in skillet.

6. Add 2 tsp. vegetable stock along with cumin, and sauté for 2 more minutes in skillet.

7. Mix sautéed vegetable with cooked quinoa and parsley.

8. Place roasted hazelnuts and sweet potato fries in a bowl. Add a little apple cider vinegar and ketchup. Serves 2.

Baked Sweet Potato Hazelnut Fries

1 sweet potato, unpeeled and sliced into thick fries or wedges
½ cup raw, skinned hazelnuts
1 garlic clove, minced

¼ tsp. dried oregano
¼ tsp. ground sage
¼ tsp. ground Himalayan pink sea salt
1 tsp. coconut oil

Directions

1. Preheat oven to 375°F.

2. Combine all ingredients, except hazelnuts, in a large bowl and mix well.

3. Spread out sweet potatoes on a baking sheet, making sure fries are not overlapping.

4. Bake for 15–20 minutes.

5. Turn oven down to 350°F.

6. Spread hazelnuts onto a baking sheet and roast for 8–10 minutes. Serves 2.

Baked Falafel with Tahini Sauce

Falafel

1¼ cups cooked garbanzo
    beans or 1 carton/tin,
    drained and rinsed

½ cup finely chopped parsley

½ sweet/Vidalia onion, chopped

2 cloves garlic, minced

1 lemon, juiced

1 tbsp. cumin

1 tbsp. gluten-free all-
    purpose flour or garbanzo
    bean/fava flour.

Pinch cayenne or chili powder

¼ tsp. ground Himalayan
    pink sea salt

Tahini Sauce

½ cup sesame tahini

½ cup warm water

3 cloves roasted garlic or
    2 cloves raw garlic

1 lemon, juiced

1 tsp. finely chopped parsley

¼ tsp. ground Himalayan
    pink sea salt

Directions

1. Heat oven 375°F.

2. Place garbanzo beans in a food processor, and pulse until
   roughly chopped.

3. Add all other ingredients, and pulse until mixed well.

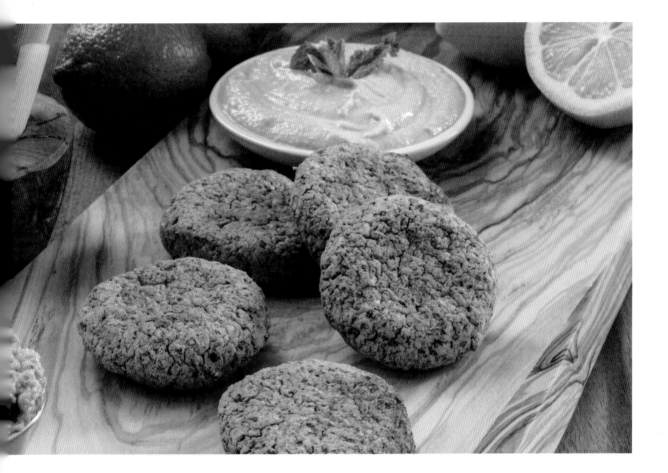

4. Line a baking sheet with unbleached parchment paper. Use an ice cream scoop to scoop mix onto parchment paper, not too close together. Should make about 8 falafels.

5. Bake for 15 minutes each side.

6. Place all tahini sauce ingredients into a food processor or blender, and run until smooth.

7. Falafel may be dipped or drizzled with Tahini sauce.

8. Serve with Parsley and Mint Salad (see recipe on page 185). Serves 2.

Vegan Meatballs

4 oz. tempeh

½ sweet onion diced finely

½ cup white mushrooms
   chopped

3 cloves garlic minced

½ tsp. dried oregano

1 tsp. vegetable stock

1 tsp. olive oil

1 tsp. coconut oil

1 tsp. tomato paste

1 tbsp. nutritional yeast

½ tsp. coconut nectar

¼ tsp. Himalayan pink salt

½ cup of gluten-free
   breadcrumbs

½ cup cashew parmesan cheese
   (see recipe on page 241)

Directions

1. Preheat oven 350°F. Place tempeh in a food processor
    and pulse until it resembles crumbles.

2. Heat a skillet over medium heat, add olive oil and onions,
    and cook for 2 minutes. Add mushrooms, garlic, oregano
    and salt and cook for 3 more minutes adding a tsp. of
    vegetable stock if it becomes too dry. Remove from
    stovetop and add mixture to tempeh, along with tomato
    paste, nutritional yeast and coconut nectar. Pulse until all
    ingredients are well mixed. Roll into 12 balls and set aside.

3. In a medium bowl mix bread crumbs and cashew
    parmesan. Transfer mixture to a large plate. Roll each
    meatball into mixture until well coated.

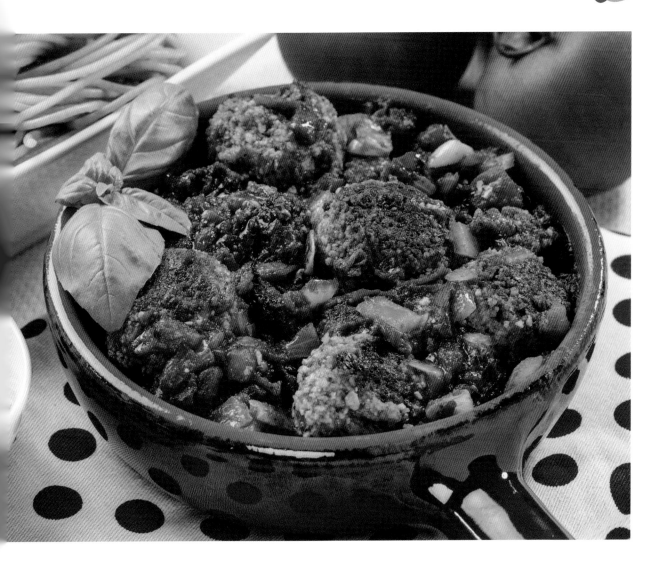

4. Heat coconut oil in a large skillet over medium high
    and cook meat balls for 2–3 minutes each side. Transfer
    meatballs to a non-stick pan or baking dish and cook in
    oven for 15–20 minutes. Serve with Sun-dried Tomato
    Marinara (see recipe on page 233) and gluten-free
    spaghetti. Top with fresh basil. Sprinkle with cashew
    parmesan cheese. Serves 2–4.

Lentil Shepherd's Pie

1 cup sprouted lentils

3¼ cups vegetable stock

1 bay leaf

1 lemon juiced

1 tsp. freshly ground herbs (mix of
    rosemary, sage and thyme)

2 lbs. russet potatoes peeled
    and chopped

3–4 carrots diced

3–4 stalks of celery diced

1 leek chopped finely

½ sweet onion diced

1 cup sliced button mushrooms

1 clove garlic minced

1 tsp. olive oil

1 tbsp. tomato paste

1 tsp. vegan Worcestershire sauce

1 tsp. coconut amino acids

1 tbsp. whole grain Dijon mustard

1 cup cashew cheese (see
    recipe on page 248)

½ tsp. Himalayan pink sea salt

¼ cup gluten-free breadcrumbs

¼ cup cashew parmesan cheese
    (see recipe on page 241)

Directions

1. Preheat oven to 350°F.

2. Place lentils, 3 cups vegetable stock and a bay leaf in a saucepan, bring to a slight boil and simmer for 30 minutes.

3. Place chopped potatoes in a saucepan covered with water, add ¼ tsp. salt, bring to a boil and cook for 20 minutes.

4. Heat a skillet over medium heat and sauté onions for 2 minutes. Add mushrooms and garlic and sauté for 2 more minutes, use a little vegetable stock if it becomes too dry. Transfer to a bowl and set aside.

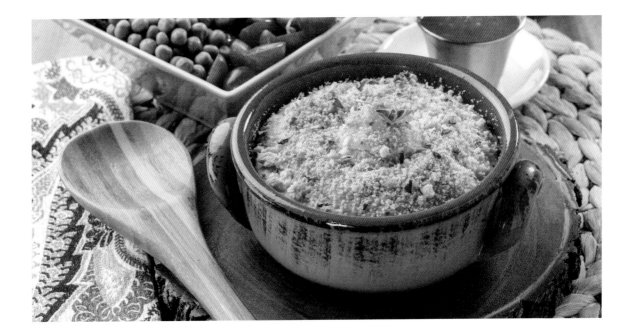

5.   In the same skillet, heat olive oil and sauté carrots, celery and leeks and fresh ground herbs add ¼ tsp. salt and cook for 3–5 minutes. Turn off heat.

6.   In a blender, place cooked onions, mushrooms and ⅓ cup of the vegetable stock from the cooked lentils, along with the Worcestershire sauce and coconut amino acids, and run until a thick gravy consistency is reached. Add this mixture to the skillet of cooked vegetables along with the cooked lentils and lemon juice, and stir all ingredients until they are well mixed.

7.   Place cooked and drained potatoes, cashew cheese, mustard and ¼ cup vegetable stock in a food processor and run on low until well mixed and smooth.

8.   Place ingredients from skillet into a ceramic or glass casserole dish and top with cashew cheese mashed potatoes.

9.   In a small bowl mix bread crumbs and cashew parmesan. Sprinkle mixture on top of the Shepherd's pie.

10. Place dish into oven and cook for 30 minutes. Serves 6.

Roasted Sweet Potatoes, Brown Basmati Rice, Chopped Parsley Salad, and Pea Tendrils

2 large sweet potatoes, washed and cut into chunks

1 cup basmati rice

2 cups vegetable stock/broth

6 shiitake mushrooms, finely chopped

4 cloves garlic, minced

1 bunch of curly parsley, washed and finely chopped

1 carrot, finely chopped

1 stalk celery, finely chopped

⅓ cucumber, finely chopped

Juice of 1 lemon

½ tsp. ground Himalayan pink sea salt

1 container of pea tendrils or sprouted greens

½ tsp. dried oregano

½ tsp. dried sage

1 tsp. olive oil

⅛ tsp. cracked black pepper

Directions

1. Preheat oven to 400°F.

2. Place rice, vegetable stock, shiitake mushrooms, and ½ the garlic in a saucepan and bring to boil. Reduce to simmer, cover, and cook for 50 minutes.

3. Place sweet potatoes, remaining garlic, olive oil, oregano, sage and ¼ tsp. salt in a large bowl and toss until coated well. Spread out on a large baking sheet and roast for 35–40 minutes.

4. Place chopped parsley, carrots, celery, and cucumber in a bowl, add lemon juice, ¼ tsp. salt, and ⅛ tsp. pepper, and toss until mixed well.

5. Serve all together, side by side, in a bowl with pea tendrils or other sprouted greens. Serves 2.

Heart-Healthy Bean Stew, Pureed Eggplant, and Red Rice

1 cup red rice

1 cup water

1½ cups cooked kidney beans or 1 tin/ can, drained and rinsed well

1½ cups cooked red beans or 1 tin/can, drained and rinsed well

2 ¾ cup vegetable stock

1 can chopped tomatoes

2 stalks celery, diced

2 carrots, diced

1 sweet/Vidalia onion diced

3 cloves garlic, minced

Juice of 1 small lime

1 tbsp. cumin

½ tsp. oregano

½ tsp. basil

1 tsp. agave or 1 tsp. coconut palm sugar

½ tsp. ground coriander

¼ tsp. ground Himalayan pink sea salt

2 bay leaves

A few basil leaves for topping

Eggplant puree (see recipe on page 211)

Directions

1. In a small saucepan, place rice, 1 cup water, ¾ cup vegetable stock, 1 minced garlic clove, and 1 bay leaf, and bring to a boil. Reduce to simmer, cover, and cook for 50 minutes.

2. Heat a large saucepan, add onion (no oil necessary), and sauté for one minute. Add celery and carrot, and sauté for 2 more minutes (add a teaspoon of vegetable stock if necessary to keep moist).

3. Add salt, cumin, coriander, bay leaf, and 2 cups of vegetable stock. Bring to a boil and reduce to simmer.

4. Add tomatoes, beans, and agave. Cover and simmer for 30 minutes.

5. Add lime juice 5 minutes before cooking ends. Top with fresh basil. Serves 4.

Eggplant Puree

1 large eggplant halved lengthwise

2 tsp. olive oil

¼ tsp. ground Himalayan pink sea salt

2 cloves of elephant garlic, unpeeled

½ lemon juiced

Directions

1. Preheat oven to 375°F.

2. Coat each half of eggplant with olive oil and salt. Place face up on a baking sheet along with unpeeled garlic and roast for 25–30 minutes until golden brown.

3. Scoop out eggplant into food processor, peel roasted garlic and add to eggplant, along with lemon juice and a pinch of ground Himalayan pink sea salt. Pulse until mixed well. Serves 2.

Red Kidney Sorghum Vindaloo

1½ cups cooked red kidney beans

1 cup cooked sorghum

1 cup of green (English) peas

½ cup cashew milk

Pinch of saffron soaked in 2 tbsp. cashew milk

2 tbsp. nutritional yeast

1 tsp. vindaloo curry powder

1 tsp. garam masala

½ sweet/Vidalia onion chopped

1 cup chopped red bell peppers

2 cloves garlic minced

1 tbsp. minced ginger root

1½ cups roasted tomatoes

1 tbsp. coconut or sesame oil

¼ tsp Himalayan pink salt

Directions

1. Heat a large skillet over medium heat and add oil. Add onion and cook for 2 minutes.

2. Add ginger, garlic and peppers and cook for 2 more minutes.

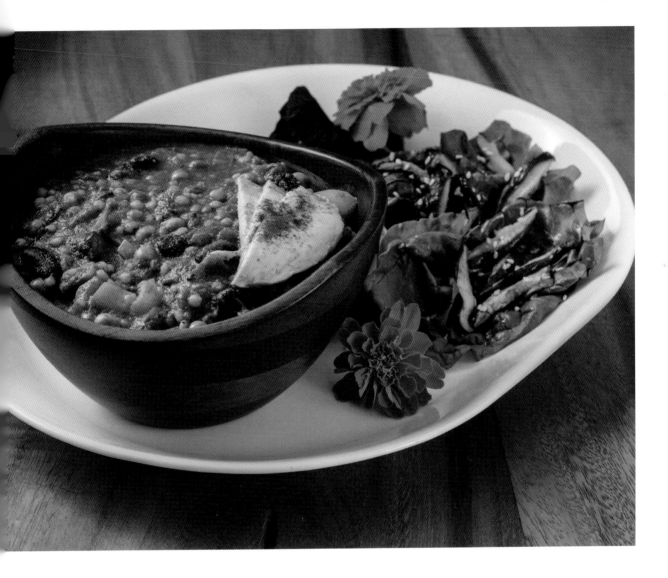

3. Add curry powder, salt, and garam masala stirring well, add tomatoes, saffron and green peas mixing well. Cook for 5 minutes.

4. Add kidney beans, sorghum, cashew milk and nutritional yeast, cook for 3 more minutes. Serves 4.

Baba Ghanoush, Watercress and Sprout Salad with Roasted Potatoes

½ cup baba ghanoush (see recipe)

2 cups watercress

1 cup sprouted greens

4 grape tomatoes, sliced

½ cup roasted potatoes (see recipe)

¼ cup pomegranate seeds

1 tbsp. sprouted pumpkin seeds

1 tsp. hemp seeds

Juice from 1 lime

Baba Ghanoush

1 large eggplant halved lengthwise

2 tsp. olive oil

¼ tsp. ground Himalayan pink sea salt

2 cloves of elephant garlic, unpeeled

1 lemon, juiced

2 tsp. sesame tahini

Roasted Potatoes

1 bag organic small yellow potatoes

1 tsp. olive oil

¼ tsp. ground sage

½ tsp. dried oregano

2 cloves garlic minced

¼ tsp. ground Himalayan pink sea salt

Directions

1. Preheat oven to 375°F.

2. Coat each half of eggplant with olive oil and salt. Place face up on a baking sheet, along with unpeeled garlic.

3. Slice potatoes in quarters and coat with garlic, olive oil, sage, oregano, and salt. Place on baking sheet with eggplant.

4. Roast eggplant and potatoes for 30 minutes until both are golden brown.

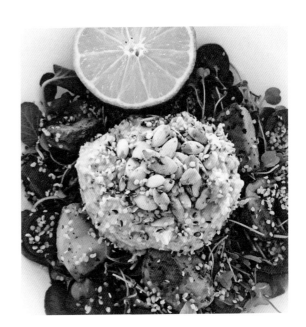

5. Scoop out eggplant into food processor, peel roasted garlic and add to eggplant, along with lemon juice, tahini, and a pinch of ground Himalayan pink sea salt. Pulse until mixed well.

6. Place watercress and sprouts in a bowl, top with tomatoes, potatoes, pomegranate seeds, hemp seeds, a large scoop of baba ghanoush, pumpkin seeds, and lime juice. Serves 2.

Hummus Arugula Spinach Salad

½ cup hummus (see recipe page on 217)

1 cup red rice chopped salad (see recipe)

1 cup arugula

1 cup spinach

¼ cup pistachios

Pinch ground Himalayan pink sea salt

Pinch cracked black pepper

Red Rice Chopped Salad

1 cup red rice

2 cup vegetable stock

1 bay leaf

2 carrots, peeled and chopped finely

2 celery stalks, chopped finely

⅓ sweet/Vidalia onion, chopped finely

½ beet, peeled and chopped finely

Juice of 1 lemon

¼ tsp. Himalayan pink salt

🕭 *Tip:* Use chopper to chop vegetables; it is quick and easy.

Hummus

1½ cups cooked garbanzo beans or
    1 tin/carton, drained and rinsed

1 lemon, juiced

1 clove garlic, minced

2 tbsp. olive oil

1 tsp. cumin

½ tsp. smoked paprika

¼ tsp. ground Himalayan
    pink sea salt

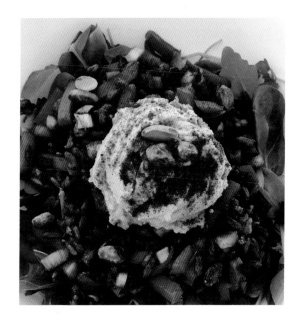

Directions

1. Place red rice, bay leaf, and vegetable stock in a saucepan and bring to a boil. Reduce to simmer and cook for 45–50 minutes. If rice was soaked overnight, it will cook in about 30–35 minutes.

2. Mix cooked rice with chopped vegetables, pistachios, lemon juice, salt, and pepper.

3. To make hummus, place all ingredients in a food processor and pulse until almost smooth. Sprinkle with smoked paprika.

4. Place arugula and spinach in a bowl, top with red rice, chopped salad, and hummus. Serves 1.

Shiitake Coriander Swiss Chard

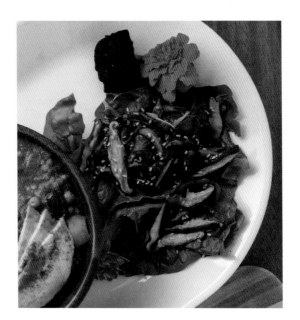

1 bunch of Swiss chard washed
    and cut horizontally into thick
    slices, large stems removed

1 cup sliced shiitake mushrooms

2 cloves of garlic minced

½ tsp. ground coriander

1 tsp. tamari sauce

1 tsp. seaweed gomasio

1 tsp. sesame oil

Directions

1. Heat a large skillet over medium heat and add sesame oil
    and shiitakes. Cook for 2 minutes.

2. Add chard, garlic, coriander, tamari and gomasio and cook for
    3–5 minutes, moving chard around in the skillet. Serves 2–4.

Spicy Green Lentil Stew

1 cup soaked green lentils,
   drained and rinsed

2 cups vegetable stock

3 carrots, finely chopped

3 stalks celery, finely chopped

1 red bell pepper, finely chopped

1 sweet/Vidalia onion,
   finely chopped

2 cloves garlic, minced

1 bay leaf

2 cups crushed tomatoes

2 presoaked sun-dried
   tomatoes, sliced thinly

1 tsp. cumin

1 tsp. chili powder

½ tsp. paprika

½ tsp. smoked paprika

¼ tsp. ground Himalayan
   pink sea salt

Juice of 1 lime

Directions

1. Place vegetable stock, lentils, bay leaf, and all other
   ingredients, except lime juice, in a medium-large
   saucepan and bring to a boil. Reduce to simmer and
   cook for 45 minutes.

2. Add lime juice just a couple of minutes before cooking
   ends. Serve with Brown Basmati Ginger Coconut Rice (see
   recipe on page 221). Serves 4.

Watercress Tendril and Lentil Salad with Lime Vinaigrette

4 cups watercress (or spinach)

2 cups pea tendrils (or other sprouted greens)

⅔ cup chopped cucumber

½ cup chopped radish

½ red onion, sliced

2 tsp. coconut or Bragg amino acids

1 cup cooked sprouted lentils

2 portobello mushrooms, sliced

Lime Vinaigrette

Juice of 1 lime

4 tbsp. olive oil

2 tbsp. fresh cilantro

2 tbsp. water

1 clove garlic

1 tsp. whole-grain Dijon mustard

1 tsp. coconut nectar

Directions

1. Place all ingredients for Lime Vinaigrette in a blender and blend until mixed well.

2. Heat a skillet over medium heat and sauté onions for 1 minute. Add amino acids and sliced mushroom, and cook until onions caramelize.

3. Place greens, cucumber, radish, lentils, mushrooms, and onions in a bowl, and top with Lime Vinaigrette.

4. Serve with Roasted Potatoes, Beets, and Carrots (see recipe on page 187). Serves 2.

Brown Basmati Ginger Coconut Rice

1 cup brown basmati rice, soaked overnight in 2
    cups vegetable stock (Do Not Drain)

1 tsp. pressed ginger juice or ½ tsp. ground ginger

½ tsp. onion powder

½ tsp. garlic granules/powder

1 bay leaf

¼ cup shredded coconut

¼ cup raisins

½ tsp. smoked paprika

⅛ tsp. salt

Directions

1. Place rice/vegetable stock mixture into a saucepan, along with ginger, onion powder, garlic powder, bay leaf, and salt, and bring to a boil. Reduce to simmer, cover, and cook for 45 minutes.

2. Take off heat, fluff up, and let sit for 5 minutes.

3. Stir in coconut, raisins, and smoked paprika. Serves 4.

Lentil Curry and Brown Rice

Lentil Curry

2 cups cooked red lentils

1 red bell pepper, sliced

½ cup sliced shiitake mushrooms

2 cloves garlic, minced

1 chunk ginger, chopped finely

⅓ cup chopped Vidalia/
    sweet onions

3 green onions, sliced

1 cup chopped tomatoes

¼ cup vegetable stock

¼ cup coconut milk

1 tbsp. curry powder

¼ tsp. ground Himalayan
    pink sea salt

¼ cup fresh, torn mint

½ tsp. coconut oil

Directions

1. Heat coconut oil in a large skillet over medium heat. Add onion and sauté for 2 minutes. Add peppers, shiitake mushrooms, green onions, garlic, and ginger, and sauté for 2 more minutes. Stir in curry powder and salt. Add tomatoes, vegetable stock, lentils, and coconut milk. Bring to a slight boil and simmer for 5–10 minutes.

2. Top with torn mint and serve with Brown Rice (see recipe on page 223). Serves 4.

Brown Rice

1 cup of brown basmati
   or short-grain rice

1 cup vegetable stock

1 cup filtered water

1 bay leaf

3 shiitake mushrooms,
   chopped finely

1 small chunk of ginger, pressed

½ tsp. garlic granules/powder

½ tsp. onion powder

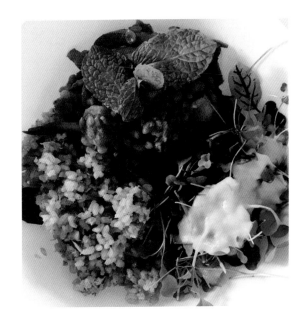

Directions

1. Place all ingredients in a saucepan and bring to a boil.
    Cover and simmer for 45 minutes. Serves 4.

Butter Bean Curry and Sprouted Brown Rice

1½ cups cooked butter/lima
    beans or 1 tin/carton
    drained and rinsed

½ tin sweet potato puree
    or 1 sweet potato,
    cooked and mashed

½ sweet onion, chopped

2 cloves garlic, minced

1 tbsp. curry powder

1 tsp. cumin

¼ tsp. nutmeg

1 carton tomato sauce or
    chopped tomatoes

1 cup frozen peas

1 cup diced carrots

1 bay leaf

1 cup sprouted brown rice

1 cup water

¾ cup vegetable stock
    (if using unsprouted brown
    rice, 1 cup veg stock)

½ tsp. coconut oil

¼ tsp. ground Himalayan
    pink sea salt

Directions

1. In a saucepan, combine water, vegetable stock, and rice, and bring to a boil. Reduce to simmer, cover, and cook for 45–50 minutes.

2. In a large skillet, heat coconut oil over medium high heat, add onions, and cook for 2–3 minutes.

3. Add carrots, garlic, curry powder, cumin, salt, and bay leaf, and cook for 2 minutes.

4. Stir in tomato sauce, sweet potato, and beans. Cook for another 2 minutes.

5. Add frozen peas. Reduce to simmer and cook for 5 more minutes. Serve with the rice. Serves 2–3.

Sorghum Salad with Navy Bean Hummus

1 cup cooked sorghum

8 cherry tomatoes, quartered

4 green onions/scallions,
    chopped

½ cup chopped cucumber

2 lemons juiced

1 tsp. olive oil

½ tsp. ground Himalayan
    pink sea salt

2 cups watercress

1 cup microgreens/
    sprouted greens

1 tsp. hemp seeds

1½ cup cooked navy beans
    or 1 tin/carton, drained
    and rinsed well

1–2 cloves of garlic, minced

1 tsp. cumin

½ tsp. smoked paprika

1 tsp. sprouted pumpkin seeds

⅛ tsp. ground Himalayan
    pink sea salt

Directions

1. Place sorghum, tomatoes, scallions, and cucumber in a bowl. Add olive oil, ½ the lemon juice, and ½ the salt and mix well. Set this sorghum mixture aside.

2. Place beans, garlic, cumin, remaining lemon juice, and salt in a food processor and pulse until almost smooth.

3. Place watercress, microgreens, and sorghum mixture into a bowl and top with hummus, smoked paprika, sprouted pumpkin seeds, and hemp seeds. You can also place in two separate bowls or plates. Serves 2.

Dry Pigeon Pea and Pomegranate Salad

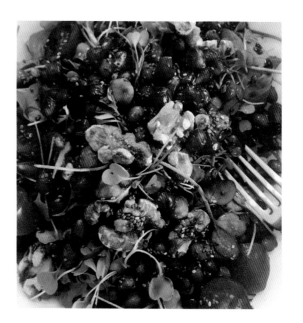

2 cups microgreens, sprouted greens, or other greens of your choice

1 cup dry pigeon peas, cooked, or ⅔ tin, drained and rinsed well

½ cup raw, unsalted walnuts

½ cup pomegranate seeds

½ cup grape or cherry tomatoes, halved

1 tsp. chia seeds

Salt and pepper to taste

Directions

1. Preheat oven to 350°F.

2. Spread walnuts out on a baking sheet and roast for 8–10 minutes.

3. Separate all ingredients evenly into 2 bowls or plates and add roasted walnuts. Top with Sweet Balsamic Vinaigrette (see recipe on page 247). Serves 2.

Sorghum and Red Kidney Bean Curried Stew

1 cup cooked sorghum

1 cup cooked red kidney
    beans or ⅔ tin, drained
    and rinsed well

½ sweet/Vidalia onion, chopped

1–2 cloves garlic, minced

Small chunk ginger,
    finely chopped

Juice of 1 lime

2 carrots, diced

2 stalks celery, diced

½ red bell pepper, diced

½ tin chopped tomatoes

⅓ cup coconut milk

¼ cup vegetable stock

1 tsp. curry powder

½ tsp. cumin

½ tsp. coriander

½ tsp. coconut oil

1 bay leaf

¼ tsp. nutmeg

¼ tsp. ground Himalayan
    pink sea salt

Directions

1. Heat a large skillet over medium-high heat and add coconut oil.

2. Add onions and sauté for 2 minutes.

3. Add carrots, celery, red peppers, bay leaf, and salt and sauté for 3 more minutes. Add a little vegetable stock to prevent vegetables from drying out.

4. Add garlic, ginger, curry powder, cumin, nutmeg, and coriander. Stir to mix and cook for another 2 minutes. Reduce to medium low and stir in coconut milk and the rest of the vegetable stock, tomatoes, kidney beans, sorghum, and lime juice.

5. Cook for 10 more minutes and serve. Serves 2. Suggested accompaniment: serve with microgreens and creamy avocado dressing (see recipe on page 251).

Turmeric Ginger Quinoa Chopped Salad

1 cup quinoa

2 cups vegetable stock

1 piece of turmeric root, peeled
    (or ½ tsp. powder)

1 chunk ginger root, peeled
    (or ½ tsp. powder)

1 bay leaf

1 clove garlic, pressed

½ tsp. onion powder

1 cup chopped romaine lettuce

½ cup chopped parsley

1 cup diced carrots

1 cup diced celery or fennel

⅓ cup diced sweet/Vidalia onion

¼ cup diced radish

½ cup cherry or grape
    tomatoes, halved

1 cup hummus (see recipe
    on page 239)

½ tsp. smoked paprika

¼ cup roasted pistachios

¼ cup roasted walnuts

1 tsp. hemp seeds

1 lemon, juiced

Pinch round Himalayan
    pink sea salt

½ tsp. smokey turmeric

½ cup diced beets

Directions

1. Place vegetable stock, quinoa, bay leaf, garlic, and onion powder into a saucepan and bring to boil. Reduce to simmer, cover, and cook for 15 minutes.

2. Cut ginger and turmeric into pieces small enough to fit into garlic press, and press out juice, add to chopped vegetables (carrots, beets, celery or fennel, radish, and onion), and set aside.

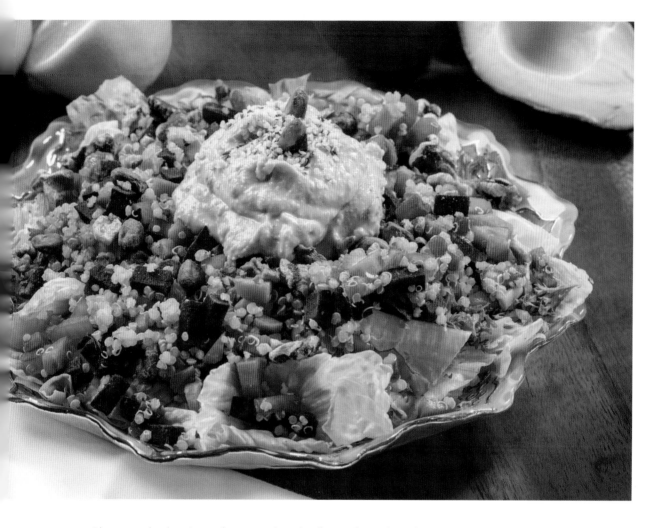

3. Place cooked quinoa (remove bay leaf) in a large bowl, add chopped vegetables, smokey turmeric, salt, and lemon juice, and mix well.

4. Place romaine and parsley into 2 separate bowls and top both with quinoa mixture, hummus, and tomatoes.

5. Sprinkle hummus with smoked paprika, roasted nuts, and hemp seeds. Serves 2.

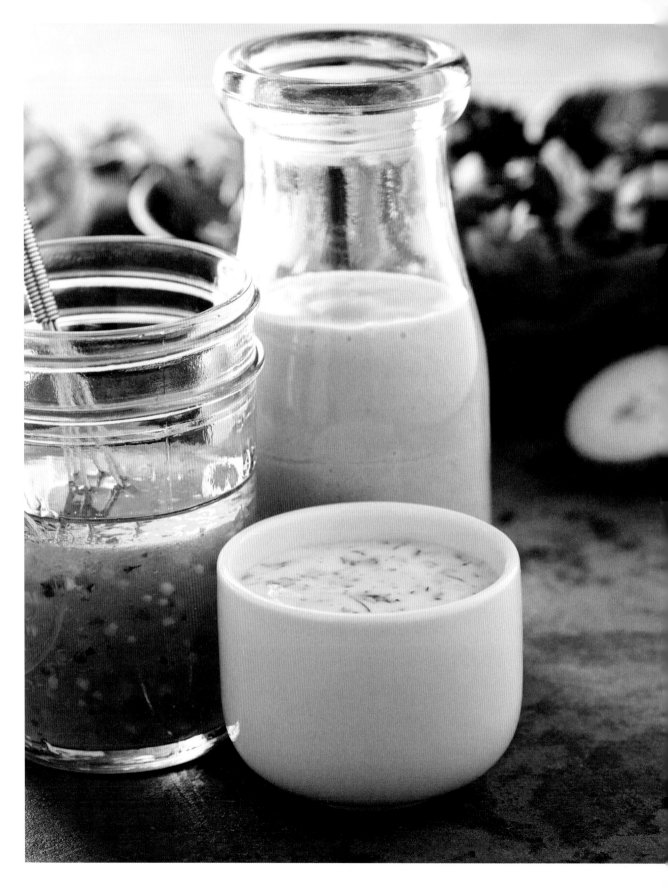

Dressings, Sauces, and Toppings

Making your own vegetable stock and dressings gives you complete control over what ingredients you are consuming. Most stocks and dressings contain canola and/or sunflower/safflower oils, which are unnecessary, unhealthy fillers. Some stocks even contain monosodium glutamate, usually hidden under different names (see excitotoxins). Using fresh vegetable juice in your stock increases nutrient content substantially and increases flavor, without the need for unhealthy additives and oils.

Oil-free Vegetable Stock

6 carrots, juiced

6 celery stalks, juiced

Handful parsley, juiced

4 cups filtered water

Juice of 1 lemon

1 tsp. onion powder

1 tsp. garlic powder

½ tsp. ground Himalayan pink sea salt

1 bay leaf

½ tsp. dried oregano

¼ tsp. dried thyme

¼ tsp. dried sage

Directions

1. Place all ingredients in a saucepan and bring to a slight boil. Reduce to simmer for 10–15 minutes.

2. Allow to cool and transfer to a jar. May be stored refrigerated for up to 1 week.

Marinara Sauce

1 large can/carton
　　crushed tomatoes

2 garlic cloves, minced

1 tbsp. olive oil

1 bay leaf

2 tbsp. ground fresh oregano

½ cup shredded fresh basil

¼ tsp. ground Himalayan
　　pink sea salt

Directions

1. Heat olive oil in a large
   skillet over medium heat.

2. Add garlic and cook for 1
   minute.

3. Add tomatoes and bay leaf,
   and bring to a slight boil.
   Reduce heat, add salt and
   oregano, and simmer for 10
   minutes.

4. Add basil just before serving.
   Serves 3–4.

Sun-dried Tomato Marinara

½ cup sun-dried tomatoes, pre-
　　soaked in warm water for 30
　　minutes prior to blending

2 cloves garlic, minced

1 tin/can fire-roasted tomatoes

1 tbsp. balsamic vinegar

1 tbsp. hemp oil or olive
　　oil (optional)

1 tsp. fresh or ½ tsp. dried thyme

1 tsp. dried oregano

Pinch ground Himalayan
　　pink sea salt

Directions

1. Place all ingredients in a
   blender or food processor
   and blend/pulse until
   mixed well.

2. Heat on stovetop or use as a
   pizza sauce. Serves 2–4.

Tomato Sauce/Salad Dressing

1 cup tomatoes, chopped

1 tsp. olive oil

1 tsp. roasted, chopped garlic

¼ tsp. dried basil (2 tbsp. fresh)

1 heaped tsp. whole-grain Dijon mustard

1 small date or ½ medjool date, pitted

1 tsp. apple cider vinegar

Pinch ground Himalayan pink sea salt

Tip: If you have some bruised tomatoes in your refrigerator, don't throw them out. You can use them in this simple recipe for Tomato Sauce/Salad Dressing:

Directions

1. Heat oil in skillet over medium heat and sauté tomatoes until very soft, about 1 minute.

2. Place in a blender along with all other ingredients and blend until smooth. May be stored in refrigerator for up to 1 week.

Ketchup

1 can/tin diced tomatoes, drained well

½ tsp. dried basil

½ tsp. garlic powder

½ tsp. oregano

1 tbsp. agave

1 tbsp. coconut nectar

2 tbsp. apple cider vinegar

Directions

1. Place all ingredients in a blender or food processor and pulse until desired consistency is obtained. If you wish to thicken mixture, add a little arrowroot.

Walnut Tofu Ricotta

1 cup soaked walnuts drained and rinsed

1 block extra firm organic tofu

2–3 cloves garlic

¼ cup nutritional yeast

¼ tsp. Himalayan pink salt

Juice of 1 lemon

Directions

1. Place all ingredients into a food processor and pulse until desired consistency is reached.

🦋 *Tip:* For a tomato ricotta cheese add 3-4 soaked and drained sun-dried tomatoes to the above ingredients.

Mango Salsa

1 cup fresh mango, diced

½ cup of cherry or grape
tomatoes, quartered

½ cup diced cucumber

⅓ cup diced sweet onion

1 lime, juiced

1 small jalapeño pepper, chopped
finely (optional)

¼ cup finely chopped cilantro

Pinch ground Himalayan pink sea salt

Directions

1. Place all ingredients in a
bowl and mix well.

Apricot Chutney

½ cup finely chopped dried apricots

Juice of 1 orange

2 tbsp. coconut palm sugar

½ sweet/Vidalia onion, finely
chopped

¼ cup raisins

½ tsp. turmeric

½ tsp. cinnamon or 1 cinnamon stick

¼ tsp. chili powder

½ tsp. whole-grain Dijon mustard

Directions

1. Place all ingredients in a
saucepan and bring to a slight
boil, reduce to simmer, and
cook for 10–15 minutes until
mixture thickens. Serves 4. Use
to top burgers, millet veggie
cakes and balls, and even
breakfast bowls.

Cranberry Sauce

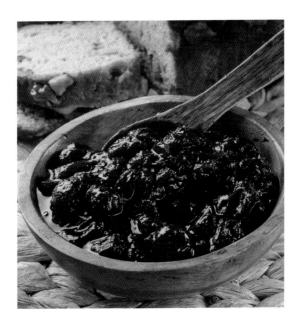

1 bag (12 oz.) fresh or
   frozen cranberries

Juice of 1 orange

1 tbsp. orange zest

¾ cup coconut palm sugar

1 tsp. cinnamon or 1 cinnamon stick

¼ tsp. cloves

Directions

1. Heat orange juice in a pan over medium heat and stir in
   coconut sugar until in melts. Add cranberries, bring to
   a slight boil, stir in cinnamon, cloves and zest, lower to
   simmer and cook for 10 minutes until cranberries start
   to pop and thicken. Serve as a sauce, jam or topping for
   savory and sweet dishes.

Smokey Turmeric Cashew Cheddar

1½ cups raw unsalted cashews

½ cup nutritional yeast

1 tsp. smokey turmeric

1 tsp. coconut nectar

½ tsp. smoked paprika

¼ tsp. cayenne

¼ tsp. Himalayan pink salt

Juice of 1 lemon

1 large clove garlic peeled or
    ½ tsp. garlic powder

¾ cup water

Directions

1. Place all ingredients in a blender and run on high until smooth and creamy. May be heated and used as a delicious sauce on pasta. Or made into a firmer cashew cheddar by the following method.

¾ cup water

1 tbsp. agar agar

Directions

1. Heat water in a saucepan on the stovetop. Add agar agar and simmer for 3–5 minutes until completely dissolved. Stir in ingredients from the blender. Transfer to a rectangle loaf pan, allow to cool, and refrigerate for 2–4 hours. Enjoy sliced on cumin curry crackers (see recipe on page 262) or use to top veggie burgers.

Hummus

1½ cups cooked garbanzo
   beans (chickpeas) or 1 can/
   tin drained and rinsed

1 lemon juiced

½ tsp. ground cumin

1 clove garlic peeled

2 tbsp. olive oil (optional)

¼ tsp. Himalayan pink salt

Directions

1. Place all ingredients in a
   food processor and pulse
   until desired consistency is
   reached. Serves 2–4.

Pumpkin Seed Hummus

3 cups cooked garbanzo
   beans or 2 cartons/tins,
   drained and rinsed well

2 limes, juiced

½ lemon, juiced

1 clove garlic, peeled

1 tbsp. raw, unsalted pumpkin
   seed butter (see resources)

1 tbsp. sesame tahini

1 tsp. cumin

½ tsp. smoked paprika

¼ tsp. allspice

⅛ tsp. nutmeg

1 tsp. coconut nectar

¼ tsp. ground Himalayan
   pink sea salt

Directions

1. Place all ingredients in a
   food processor and pulse
   until almost smooth.
   Serves 4.

Smokey Butter Bean Tahini Pâté

¾ cup cooked butter beans or ½ tin/can
   drained and rinsed well

2 tbsp. ground sesame seeds

½ lemon, juiced

1 clove garlic, minced

1 tsp. olive oil

¼ tsp. smoked paprika

⅛ tsp. ground Himalayan pink sea salt

Directions

1. Place all ingredients in a food processor and pulse until almost smooth.

2. Top with extra smoked paprika and serve on gluten-free toast, topped with slices of fresh tomato. Serves 1–2.

Great Northern Bean and Beet Hummus

1½ cups cooked great northern
    beans or 1 tin/can,
    drained and rinsed well

Juice of 1 lemon

1 garlic clove, pressed or minced

2 tbsp. raw beets, diced finely

1 tbsp. sprouted pumpkin seeds

1 tbsp. olive oil (optional)

1 tsp. cumin

⅛ tsp. ground Himalayan
    pink sea salt

Directions

1. Place all ingredients in a food processor and pulse until desired consistency is reached. Serves 2–4.

Cashew Parmesan Cheese

1 cup raw unsalted cashews

4 tbsp. nutritional yeast

½ tsp. garlic powder

¼ tsp. salt

Directions

1. Place all ingredients in a food processor and run on low until it resembles parmesan cheese.

Tahini Coleslaw Dressing

3 tbsp. sesame tahini

½ lemon, juiced

2 tbsp. water

1 tbsp. whole-grain Dijon mustard

1 tbsp. apple cider vinegar

1 tbsp. nutritional yeast

2 tsp. coconut palm sugar

Pinch ground Himalayan pink sea salt

Pinch freshly cracked pepper

> **Tip:** **Red Cabbage Slaw**: Combine 4 cups finely chopped red cabbage with 2 cups grated carrots and ½ cup finely chopped onion. Mix well with Tahini Coleslaw Dressing.

Directions

1. Place all in ingredients in a small bowl or measuring jug, and whisk until well blended.

2. The mustard seeds will still be whole, which adds texture.

Simple Guacamole

1 avocado,

½ lime juiced

1 tsp. cumin

¼ tsp. ground Himalayan
    pink sea salt

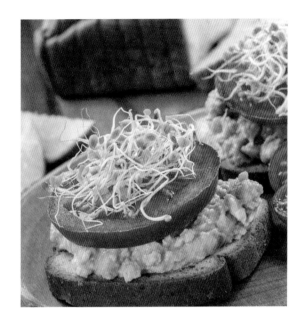

Directions

1. Slice avocado in half, remove stone, and scoop flesh into
    a small bowl.

2. Add lime juice, cumin, and salt and mash. Mix well with
    a fork. Serve on gluten-free toast that has been coated
    with a little coconut oil and fresh pressed garlic, or if you
    prefer to use no oil just rub a little raw garlic over toast
    before topping with guacamole. Serves 2.

Mango Lime Dressing

½ cup mango chunks,
    fresh or frozen

2 tbsp. water

Zest of 1 lime

2 limes, juiced

1 medjool date, pit removed

1 tbsp. hemp oil or olive oil

Directions

1. Place ingredients in blender and blend until smooth.

Miso Ginger Dressing

1 tsp. organic sweet
    white miso paste

1 tsp. grated fresh ginger

1 carrot, grated

¼ cup hemp oil

¼ cup apple cider vinegar

Directions

1. Place all ingredients in a blender and blend until smooth.

Miso Mushroom Gravy

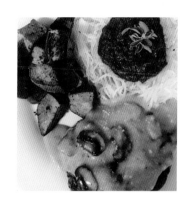

3 cups vegetable stock

1 cup sliced white or baby Portobello
    mushrooms

2 tbsp. water

2 tbsp. sweet white miso

¼ cup ground gluten-free whole oats or
    oat flour

1 tbsp. low-sodium tamari sauce

1 tbsp. nutritional yeast

1 tbsp. cacao butter

½ tsp. onion powder

1 tsp. sesame oil

2 tbsp. arrowroot for thickening

Cracked black pepper to taste

Directions

1. Heat skillet over medium heat and add sesame oil.

2. Add mushrooms, cook for 3 minutes, and set aside.

3. In a small bowl, whisk together miso and water until well blended, and set aside.

4. In a saucepan, heat cacao butter over medium heat.

5. Stir in oat flour until smooth, slowly wisk in vegetable stock and miso mixture, stir well.

6. Whisk in onion powder, nutritional yeast, and tamari sauce.

7. Mix arrowroot with a little water and slowly add to sauce, whisking until it starts to thicken to desired consistency.

8. Stir in mushrooms and serve. Serves 4–6. Use to top pasta, burgers, lentil loaf, potatoes, and vegetables.

Eggplant Puree

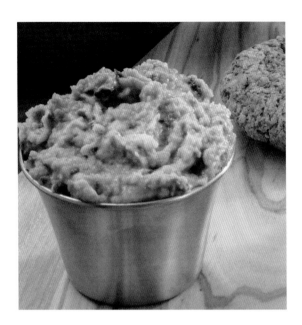

1 large eggplant halved lengthwise

2 tsp. olive oil

¼ tsp. ground Himalayan
   pink sea salt

2 cloves of elephant garlic, unpeeled

½ lemon, juiced

Directions

1. Preheat oven to 375°F.

2. Coat each half of eggplant with olive oil and salt.

3. Place face up on a baking sheet along with unpeeled garlic and roast for 25–30 minutes until golden brown.

4. Scoop out eggplant into food processor, peel roasted garlic and add to eggplant along with lemon juice and a pinch of ground Himalayan pink sea salt.

5. Pulse until mixed well. Serves 2.

❀ *Tip:* Smokey Baba Ganoush: follow recipe above for Eggplant Puree, adding 2 tsp. sesame tahini to the ingredients in the food processor and sprinkle with smoked paprika.

Cilantro Lime Vinaigrette

Juice of 1 lime

4 tbsp. olive oil

2 tbsp. fresh cilantro

2 tbsp. water

1 tsp. whole-grain Dijon mustard

1 tsp. coconut nectar

1 clove garlic

Pinch ground Himalayan
pink sea salt

Pinch cracked black pepper

Direction

1. Use blender to blend all ingredients well. Serves 4.

Sweet Balsamic Vinaigrette

2 tbsp. hemp oil or olive oil

2 tsp. Dijon mustard

2 tbsp. balsamic vinegar

1 tsp. coconut nectar or agave

Directions

1. Place all ingredients in a blender and blend until smooth. Serves 2.

Cashew Cheese

1 cup soaked raw, unsalted
    cashews, drained and rinsed

1 lemon, juiced

3 tbsp. water

2 tbsp. nutritional yeast

1 tsp. coconut or Bragg
    amino acids

½ tsp. garlic powder

¼ tsp. ground Himalayan
    pink sea salt

¼ tsp. ground black pepper

Directions

1. Place all ingredients except
   water in a food processor,
   and pulse until mixed well.

2. Turn power on low and
   slowly add the water until
   consistency is smooth.

3. Add more water if needed
   to reach desired consistency.
   Serves 4.

Hemp Mayonnaise

3 tbsp. hemp oil or olive oil

1 cup hemp seeds

½ lemon, juiced

½ tsp. ground Himalayan
    pink sea salt

2 tsp. onion powder or 1
    tbsp. finely chopped
    sweet/Vidalia onion

1 tbsp. apple cider vinegar

½ tsp. agave

¼ cup filtered water

Directions

1. Blend all ingredients except
   water, add water slowly
   until desired thickness is
   achieved. Serves 3–4.

Tahini Cheese

2 tbsp. sesame tahini

Juice of 1 lemon

1 tsp. nutritional yeast

½ tsp. garlic powder

⅛ tsp. turmeric

⅛ tsp. ground Himalayan
    pink sea salt

1 to 2 tbsp. filtered water

Pepper to taste

Directions

1. Place tahini in a bowl and stir in lemon juice until it thickens. Place tahini mix into a food processor along with nutritional yeast, garlic powder, turmeric and salt and pulse until well mixed.

2. Add water until desired consistency is achieved. Pepper to taste. Serves 2.

Peanut Lime and Coconut Dressing

2 limes, juiced

1 heaped tbsp. smooth
    peanut butter

¼ cup coconut milk

1 tbsp. hemp seeds

1 tbsp. rice vinegar

1 tsp. sesame oil

1 tsp. agave or coconut nectar

½ tsp. smoked paprika (optional)

Pinch ground Himalayan
    pink sea salt

Directions

1. Place all ingredients in a blender and blend until smooth. Add water if necessary. Serves 2.

Lemon Garlic Herb Vinaigrette

1 tbsp. freshly ground mix of
    rosemary, sage and thyme

1–2 garlic cloves minced

Juice of 2 lemons

¼ cup olive oil

⅛ tsp. pink Himalayan sea salt

Directions

1. Place all ingredients in a jar, secure lid and shake until well mixed. Serves 2–4.

Lemon Banana Pumpkin Seed Cream

1 lemon, juiced

1 banana

2 medjool dates, pitted

1 tbsp. sprouted pumpkin seeds or
    soaked raw pumpkin seeds

2 tbsp. hemp seeds

Directions

1. Place all ingredients in a food processor and pulse until smooth.

2. Add a little plant milk if necessary to achieve desired consistency.

3. Enjoy as an energy pudding or as topping on a breakfast bowl, pancakes, or muffins. May be stored refrigerated up to 3 days. Serves 1.

Tahini Lime Banana Cream

1 banana

1 tbsp. tahini

Juice of 1 lime

2 tbsp. hemp seeds

½ tsp. maca

2 tsp. coconut nectar

Directions

1. Place all ingredients in a food processor and pulse until smooth.

2. Use to top breakfast bowls, muffins, breads, or enjoy alone. Serves 1.

Creamy Avocado Dressing (oil free)

½ avocado

Juice of 1 large lime

1 tbsp. hemp seeds

1 tbsp. rice vinegar

3 tbsp. water

2 tsp. agave or 2 medjool dates, pitted

¼ tsp. ground Himalayan pink sea salt

Direction

1. Blend all ingredients until smooth and creamy. Serves 1–2.

Smokey Cashew Cheese Sauce

Juice of 1 lemon

½ cup soaked cashews
    drained and rinsed

2 tbsp. plant milk

2 heaped tbsp. nutritional yeast

½ tsp. onion powder

½ tsp. garlic powder

¼ tsp. smoked paprika

Pinch pink Himalayan sea salt

Direction

1. Place all ingredients in a food processor and run on low until smooth. Heat on stovetop until sauce thickens, use to top pasta, burgers and vegetables. Serves 2.

Avocado Mayonnaise (oil free)

½ avocado

1 large lime, juiced

1 tbsp. rice vinegar

1 tbsp. hemp seeds

½ tsp. onion powder

½ tsp. garlic powder

3 tbsp. water

¼ tsp. ground Himalayan
    pink sea salt

1 tsp. agave

Directions

1. Place ingredients in a blender or food processor and mix until thick and creamy. Serves 1–2.

Coconut Cheese Sauce

½ cup light coconut milk

2 tbsp. nutritional yeast

1 tsp. sweet white miso

½ tsp. onion powder

½ tsp. garlic powder

½ tsp. arrowroot to
    thicken if necessary

Directions

1. Place all ingredients in a jug
   or small bowl and whisk
   until smooth.

2. Heat on stovetop over
   medium low until thickens.
   Serves 2.

Barbecue Sauce

½ cup tomato paste

⅓ cup unsweetened applesauce

¼ cup coconut nectar

1 tbsp. coconut amino acids

1 tbsp. vegan Worcestershire sauce

1 tbsp. whole grain Dijon mustard

1 tbsp. apple cider vinegar

⅛ tsp. cayenne

1 tsp. chilli powder

1 tsp. smoked paprika

1 tbsp. garlic paste

1 tbsp. minced ginger

¼ tsp. black pepper

½ tsp. onion powder

Directions

1. Place all ingredients in a food
   processor or blender and run
   until smooth or until desired
   consistency is reached. Makes
   about 1 cup. Store refrigerated
   for up to 1 week.

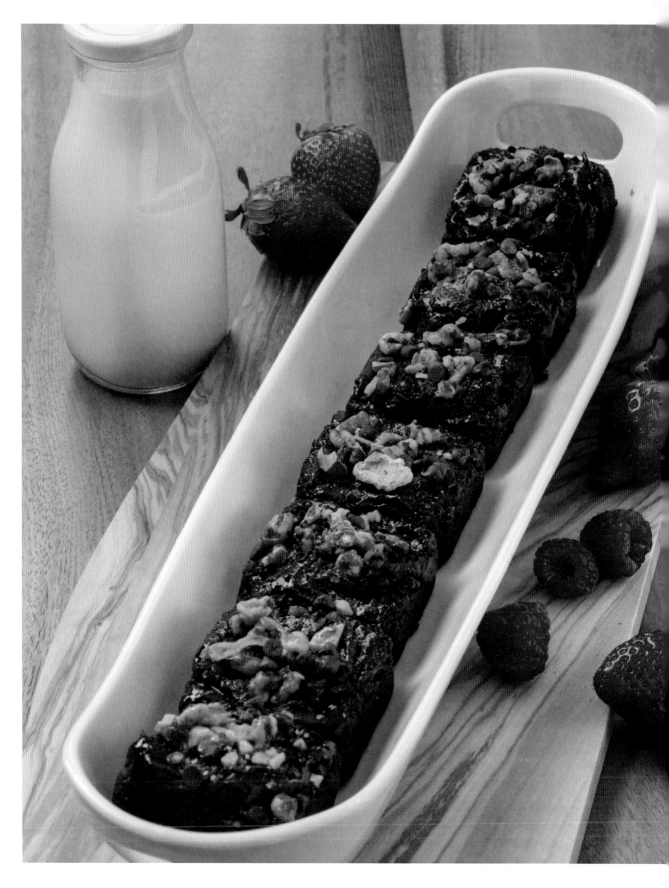

Snacks

Although fresh fruit, vegetables, nuts, and seeds by themselves are amazing powerhouse snacks, occasionally we may feel the need to reach for something a little different. In this section, you will find some of my favorite snacks. Prepare a batch in advance so you have healthy bites always available. My homemade bars are loaded with superfoods and provide long-lasting high energy. Find them in my Live bars section on page 147. They are great as a snack on the go or when you may be too busy to stop and eat a full meal.

Chocolate Chip Cookies

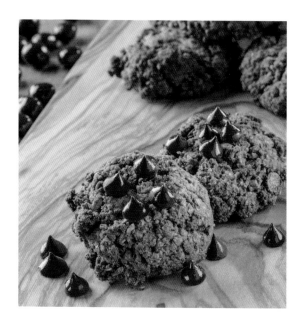

1 cup quick cooking gluten-free oats

½ cup coconut flour

1 cup coconut palm sugar

½ cup melted cacao butter

½ cup vegan chocolate chips

¼ cup unsweetened hemp
    or almond milk

1 tsp. vanilla extract

½ tsp. baking soda

½ tsp. ground Himalayan pink salt

Directions

1. Preheat oven 350°F. Place sugar, salt and melted cacao butter in large bowl and mix well. Add plant milk and vanilla extract mixing well.

2. In separate bowl mix flours and baking soda, and add slowly to the wet ingredients without overmixing. Fold in chocolate chips, and allow mixture to sit for 15 minutes.

3. Using an ice cream scoop place each scoop on non-stick baking sheet or line with unbleached parchment paper. Makes about 12 good size cookies. Bake for 15–20 minutes.

Banana Energy Balls

1 banana
½ cup cooked quinoa
4 large medjool dates, chopped
½ cup raw pecans, chopped
2 tsp. cinnamon
¼ tsp. nutmeg
½ tsp. maca
2 tbsp. coconut shreds

Directions

1. Place all ingredients, except coconut, in food processor and pulse until mixed well.

1. Roll mixture into 10 balls, then roll balls in coconut shreds. May be stored in refrigerator for up to 5 days.

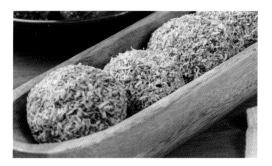

Lemon Banana Chia Pudding

1 banana
¾ cup almond milk
Juice of 1 lemon
2 medjool dates, pitted
2 tbsp. hemp seeds
¼ tsp. maca root powder
¼ cup chia seeds

Directions

1. Place all ingredients in a food processor or blender on low until mixed well.

2. Transfer to a jar or short glass, cover, and refrigerate for at least 4 hours, preferably overnight. Serves 1.

Hazelnut Truffles

2 cups raw skinned hazelnuts

10 medjool dates pitted

1 tbsp. cacao powder

6 oz. vegan dark chocolate roughly chopped

1 tbsp. cacao butter

¼ cup shredded coconut

¼ tsp. Himalayan Pink salt

Directions

1. Preheat oven to 300°F. Spread hazelnuts out onto a baking sheet and roast for 10 minutes. Remove and set aside to cool for 5 minutes.

2. Place hazelnuts in a food processor and pulse until they resemble bread crumbs. Place into a bowl and set aside.

3. Place dates into food processor and pulse until they form a ball. Add half the hazelnut meal and ⅛ tsp. salt, and pulse until well mixed. Place ⅓ cup of hazelnut meal aside, and continue to add the remainder to the food processor as you pulse until it resembles a loose dough mixture. Roll mixture into balls using your hands. Makes 12–15 balls depending on size. Place balls on a baking

sheet lined with unbleached parchment paper and place in the freezer.

4. Heat water in a kettle until almost boiling and add 4 cups of the hot water to a saucepan. Take a small heat proof bowl and place it in the saucepan, it is fine if the bowl touches the water, and add chopped chocolate. It should take no more than 1–2 minutes to melt.

5. In a separate saucepan add cacao butter and heat gently until it melts. Add it to melted chocolate mixing well.

6. Remove balls from freezer and dip into melted chocolate/ cacao butter one at a time, remove with fork and place back onto the parchment paper lined baking sheet, sprinkle with a little almond meal, coconut and salt. Place balls into refrigerator for at least 30 minutes.

Cashew, Coconut Yogurt Cream

½ cup presoaked cashews, drained and rinsed

2 tbsp. hemp seeds

1 banana

1 unsweetened coconut yogurt

1 lemon juiced

4 medjool dates, pitted

½ tsp. vanilla extract

¼ tsp. cinnamon

Directions

1. Place all ingredients in a food processor and pulse or process on low until smooth.

2. Eat as an energy snack or use to top breakfast bowls or muffins. A good source of plant protein! May be stored refrigerated for up to 3 days. Serves 2.

Banana Pecan Cream

2 bananas

Juice of 1 lime

½ cup presoaked raw pecans

1 tsp. raw sesame seeds

4 medjool dates, pitted

1 tbsp. hemp protein or 2 tbsp. hemp seeds

1 tsp. maca root powder

Directions

1. Place all ingredients in a food processor and blend on low until smooth.

2. This is a very rich snack and can be eaten alone or used to top pancakes, breakfast bowls, or spread on breakfast breads. May be stored refrigerated for up to 3 days. Serves 2.

Black Bean Brownies

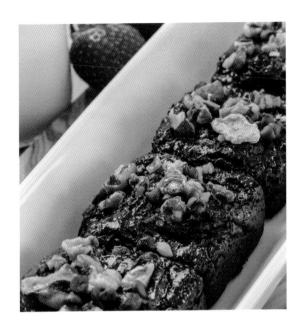

3 cups cooked black beans
  or 2 cans/cartons black
  beans drained and rinsed

2 chia eggs (2 heaped tbsp.
  ground chia seeds mixed
  well with 6 tbsp. plant milk)

1½ cups raw cacao powder

2 cups coconut palm sugar

3 tbsp. melted coconut oil

2 tsp. vanilla extract

½ tsp. pink Himalayan sea salt

3 tsp. baking powder

½ cup raw or toasted walnuts

½ cup vegan semi-sweet
  chocolate chips

Directions

1. Preheat oven to 350°F. With the exception of the
    walnuts and half of the chocolate chips, place all
    ingredients in a food processor, and pulse until well
    mixed.

2. Place mixture in a muffin pan or mini loaf pan, and top
    with a few chocolate chips and walnuts. Bake muffins for
    25 minutes or mini loaves for 35 minutes. Allow to cool
    before removing from pan. Makes 16 muffins or 10 mini
    loaves.

Curry Roasted Cashews

1 cup raw, unsalted cashews

1 tsp. curry powder

1 tsp. ground cumin

1 tsp. sesame oil

¼ tsp. ground Himalayan
   pink sea salt

Directions

1. Heat oven to 350°F.

2. Line a baking sheet with
   parchment paper.

3. Place the cashews into a
   bowl and add the salt, curry
   powder, cumin, and sesame
   oil, and toss to combine.

4. Spread the cashews evenly
   on the baking sheet
   and roast, until evenly
   browned, about 10 minutes.
   Serve warm or at room
   temperature. Serves 2–4.

Cumin Curry Crackers

¼ cup coconut flour

¼ cup cooked sprouted lentils

2 tbsp. balsamic vinegar

1 tsp. coconut oil

1 tsp. hemp oil

1 tbsp. nutritional yeast

1 tbsp. curry powder

1 tsp. cumin

½ tsp. coconut nectar

¼ tsp. ground Himalayan
   pink sea salt

Directions

1. Preheat oven to 300°F.

2. Place all ingredients in a food
   processor and pulse until a dough
   forms.

3. Line a baking sheet with
   unbleached parchment paper.
   Flatten or roll out dough onto
   baking sheet.

4. Bake for 30–45 minutes. Once
   cooled, break into pieces.

Kale Chips

Popped Sorghum

1 bunch of curly kale

1 tsp. olive oil

¼ tsp. ground Himalayan
   pink sea salt

½ cup sorghum grain

¼ cup nutritional yeast

1 tbsp. coconut nectar

Directions

1. Heat oven to 375°F.

2. Wash kale, tear green away
   from stalks, and throw away
   stalks.

3. Dry kale well and place in a
   large bowl.

4. Mix well with olive oil and
   salt.

5. Line a large baking sheet
   with unbleached parchment
   paper, spread kale out onto
   baking sheet, and roast for
   10 minutes until crispy.
   Serves 2–4.

Directions

1. Heat a large pot over
   medium high, and add ¼
   cup sorghum, cover with
   a lid. Shake the pot a few
   times so it does not burn.
   When there is more than
   10 seconds between pops,
   sorghum is ready. Transfer
   to a bowl and repeat
   with the other ¼ cup of
   sorghum.

2. Place popped sorghum in
   a large bowl, sprinkle with
   nutritional yeast and drizzle
   with coconut nectar.
   Serves 2.

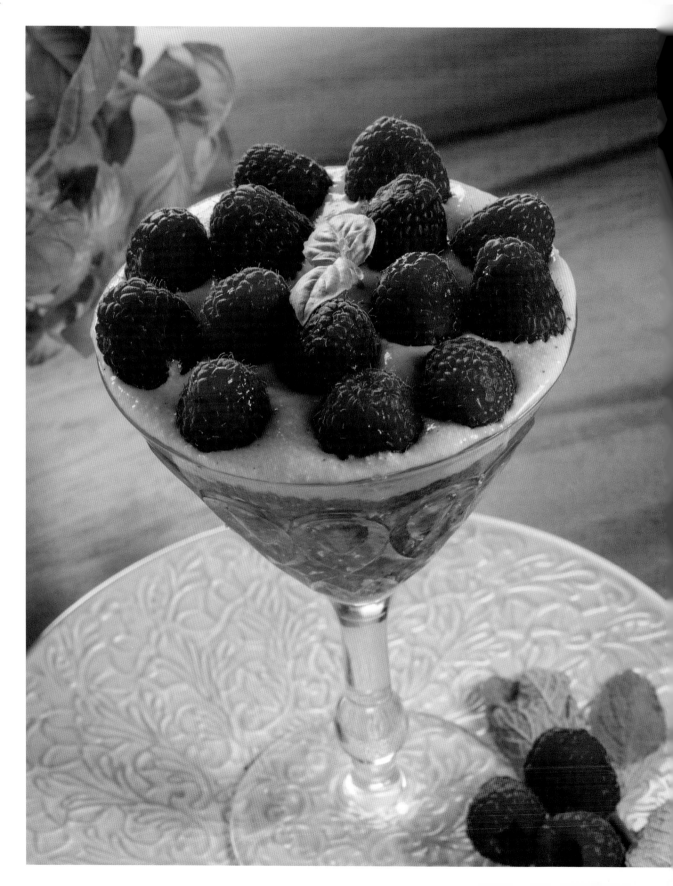

Appendix

Vitamins and Minerals

It is important to understand that vitamins and minerals are essential to proper growth and development. They are groups of beneficial micronutrient compounds naturally occurring in many different foods. Without vitamins and minerals, we would not be alive. Consuming a plant-based diet of whole foods ensures that the body will acquire an abundance of vitamins and minerals crucial to a healthy body and mind. Consuming foods in their whole form is the best way to receive vitamins and minerals. Choosing to take isolated compounds in the form of pills and supplements over a healthy plant-based diet is a big mistake.

Vitamin A

Vitamin A is very important to immune function, to vision, and to reproductive health. Vitamin A is fat soluble, and can be stored in the body for long periods of time. There is no toxicity derived from consuming foods rich in vitamin A, but there is potential toxicity when over consuming isolated vitamin A in supplement form. Plants containing vitamin A include green leafy vegetables, orange and yellow fruits and vegetables, and tomatoes.

Beta Carotene

Beta carotene is the precursor to vitamin A, when it is consumed, the body converts it into vitamin A. It is a powerful antioxidant that staves off free radicals. Beta carotene gives fruits and vegetables their yellow-orange pigment color. Beta carotene serves the same beneficial functions as vitamin A, providing a healthy immune system, skin and eye health. The best sources of beta carotene are, green leafy vegetables, and, orange and yellow fruits and vegetables.

Vitamin B1

Vitamin B1, also known as thiamine, helps the body covert carbohydrates into glucose, which is important for energy production. All B vitamins are water soluble and therefore, not stored in the body for long periods of time. Thiamine plays a crucial role in maintaining a healthy nervous system, and helps to keep the heart strong and healthy. Rich plant sources of thiamine include nutritional yeast, whole grains, and kidney beans. Other sources are asparagus, mushrooms, eggplant, potatoes, sunflowers seeds, brussel sprouts, and tomatoes. Be careful not to overcook these foods as overcooking can destroy thiamine.

Vitamin B2

Vitamin B2, also known as riboflavin, plays an important role in balancing the adrenal glands, and keeping the nervous system healthy. Riboflavin helps to maintain healthy hair and skin, and may even ward off migraine headaches. Riboflavin may also prevent free radical formation, giving it anti-cancer benefits. Good plant sources of riboflavin include whole grains, nutritional yeast, sun dried tomatoes, mushrooms, spinach, and almonds.

Vitamin B3

Vitamin B3, also called niacin, is very important to a healthy cardiovascular system. It helps to balance cholesterol levels, and assists in the regulation of blood glucose. Niacin is also very important to brain function and healthy skin. Plant sources of niacin include green peas, mushrooms, squash, pumpkin, sweet potatoes, corn, and seaweed.

Vitamin B5

Vitamin B5, also known as pantothenic acid, plays a crucial role in the metabolism of energy, by converting carbohydrates into glucose. This energy helps to increase neurotransmission in the brain to carry signals through the body, keeping it working efficiently. Pantothenic acid helps to keep the digestive system healthy, and the adrenal glands functioning optimally. Good plant sources of pantothenic acid include avocado, lentils, portobello mushrooms, broccoli, and sun-dried tomatoes.

Vitamin B6

Vitamin B6, also called pyridoxine, is important to a healthy nervous system, and a healthy metabolism. Pyridoxine also helps with mood and can ward off anxiety, depression, and PMS symptoms. Pyridoxine plays a role in the maintenance of a healthy heart and strong immune system. Good plant sources of pyridoxine include avocados, whole grains, nuts, seeds and beans.

Vitamin B12

Vitamin B12, also known as cobalamin, plays a crucial role in the formation of red blood cells, and in maintaining a healthy nervous system. B12 is not abundant in plant sources, so if you are in doubt about how much you are receiving though your diet, get your blood level checked. It is not really possible to overdose on B12, so taking a supplement is pretty harmless. Good plant sources of B12 include chlorella, seaweed, aloe vera, tempeh, miso, sauerkraut and nutritional yeast.

Biotin

Biotin, also known as B7, is part of the complex group of B vitamins. Biotin strengthens the hair, nails and skin. Biotin helps the metabolic process by converting nutrients into energy. Good plant sources of biotin include beans, whole grains, nuts, bananas, cauliflower and mushrooms.

Folate (folic acid)

Folate also called folic acid, or B9, is another B vitamin that assists the body in optimal growth, and the manufacturing of DNA. It is also important in regulating heart rhythm, and aiding in muscle repair. Folate is very important during pregnancy, and deficiency is linked to birth abnormalities. Rich plant sources of folate include leafy greens, avocado, oranges, broccoli, brussel sprouts, beans and lentils.

Vitamin C

Vitamin C, one of the most powerful antioxidant compounds that boosts immunity, wards off colds, prevents scurvy, and has anti-cancer properties. Vitamin C is also known as ascorbic acid, is water soluble, and plays a major role in collagen formation, and bone and connective tissue health. Vitamin C is abundant in the plant kingdom, great sources being citrus fruits, bell peppers, leafy greens, broccoli, berries and tomatoes.

Vitamin D

Vitamin D is a fat-soluble vitamin made up of three compounds D1, D2 and D3. Also, well known as the sunshine vitamin, because when we expose our skin to the sun we are able to manufacture vitamin D. This important nutrient regulates the absorption of calcium and phosphorus, keeping our bones strong and healthy. It also plays a vital role in the immune system, helping ward off auto-immune disease. Sunshine is the best source of vitamin D. However, there are good plant sources of vitamin D including chlorella, seaweeds, spirulina, mushrooms, hemp and tofu. Avocado, sesame oil, pumpkin seed oil, and hemp oil, help the body to store fat soluble vitamin D.

Vitamin E

Vitamin E is important to cardiovascular health by helping the body maintain beneficial cholesterol levels. It is also a powerful antioxidant which keeps cells healthy, and protects them from free radical damage. Good plant sources of vitamin E include avocado, almonds, sunflower seeds, squash, pumpkin, and dark leafy vegetables.

Vitamin K

Vitamin K is a fat-soluble vitamin that is vital to blood clotting, and helps keep bones strong and healthy. Vitamin K is abundant in green leafy vegetables, chlorella, spirulina, nori seaweed, brussel sprouts, broccoli, cabbage, and prunes. Beneficial bacteria in the intestines can also produce vitamin K.

Calcium

Calcium is the most abundant mineral found in the body, and serves many major functions. The bones and teeth store ninety-nine percent of the body's calcium. It is vital for healthy bones, muscle contraction, and regulating heart rhythm. Calcium works with vitamin D for maximum absorption. Plants rich in calcium include dark leafy greens, broccoli, almonds, sesame seeds, sunflower seeds, figs, and sweet potatoes.

Copper

Copper is a trace mineral, meaning we only need very small amounts in the diet to benefit from its functions. Although copper is found in all tissues within the body, most of it is found in the liver. Copper works in sync with iron to manufacture red blood cells, and it helps to keep the immune system functioning optimally. Copper also assists in the formation of collagen, and produces the pigment that colors hair and skin, known as melanin. Copper can be found in cashews, seeds, spinach, cremini mushrooms, tomatoes, eggplant, potatoes, and prunes.

Iodine

Iodine is an essential mineral, and vital to the proper functioning of the thyroid gland. Maintaining balance of the amount of iodine in the body is critical, too much can increase thyroid function, and too little can decrease it. Seaweed is a rich source of iodine, as is iodized salt. Other plant foods containing iodine include cranberries, navy beans, strawberries and potatoes.

Iron

Iron's main function in the body is to transport red blood cells via hemoglobin. Iron is vital to energy production in the cells, as it delivers oxygen rich blood to muscles during activity such as exercise. Iron also assists in healthy circulation and digestion. Rich sources of iron include beans, spinach, strawberries, raisins, oatmeal, peas and lentils.

Magnesium

Magnesium is a major component in the functioning of muscles and nerves. Magnesium helps to regulate heartbeat, and assists calcium in the maintenance of strong bones and teeth. Magnesium relieves constipation, helps to keep kidney stones at bay, and eases migraine headaches. Good plant sources of magnesium include whole grains, figs, green leafy vegetables, nuts, beans, and avocados.

Manganese

Manganese is important to calcium absorption, thyroid function, stabilizing blood glucose, and is a contributing factor to the metabolism of lipids and amino acids. Plant sources of manganese include garlic, oats, leafy greens, figs, bananas, turmeric, nuts, whole grains, and berries.

Molybdenum

Molybdenum is a trace mineral that plays a major role in biological functions. Molybdenum assists in the metabolism of carbohydrates and fats, and is a main player in the enzymatic breakdown of certain amino acids within the body. Beans, lentils, peas and leafy greens are good plant sources of molybdenum.

Phosphorus

Phosphorus is important to healthy bone formation, hormonal balance, and proper digestion. Phosphorus is an important component in chemical reactions, and cellular repair. It also assists in the optimal utilization of nutrients. Rich sources of phosphorus include rice, nuts, beans, sunflower seeds, pumpkin and squash.

Potassium

Potassium is an electrolyte as well as a mineral and therefore plays a major part in hydrating the body. Proper hydration is vital for energy, and optimal body function. Potassium helps to regulate heart rhythm, muscle contraction, and nerve conduction. Rich sources of potassium include bananas, sweet potatoes, white potatoes, watermelon, squash, beets, spinach and tomatoes.

Selenium

Selenium is an essential trace mineral and antioxidant. It is a major player in immune function, and protects the body from free radical damage. It works as a natural anti-inflammatory in preserving muscle tissue. Selenium is also heart protective, important in thyroid function, and may help reduce the risk of cognitive decline. Plant food sources include brown rice, walnuts, brazil nuts, and nutritional yeast.

Zinc

Zinc plays a major role in keeping the immune system healthy by regulating cell production. Zinc assists hundreds of different enzymes in the body, enabling them to function optimally. Pumpkin seeds, garbanzo beans, cashews, mushrooms, spinach and nutritional yeast are all good plant sources of zinc.

Glossary

Amino acids

Amino acids are found in protein, and are made up of a large group of organic compounds joined together via peptide bonds. Amino acids come in two forms, essential and non-essential amino acids, and these compounds play a vital role in growth and development, and in immunity.

Ancient Grains

Ancient grains are grains that have not been altered or modified in any way since they were first cultivated. Ancient grains include quinoa, millet, sorghum, amaranth, teff, chia seeds, farro, spelt, and kamut. Even though farro, spelt and kamut are not gluten-free, some people with gluten sensitivity can still tolerate them.

Antioxidants

Antioxidants are substances found in foods that protect the body's cells from free radical damage. The major micronutrients that work as antioxidants are Beta carotene, vitamin C, vitamin E and selenium. Colorful fruits and vegetables are high in antioxidants.

Chlorophyll

Chlorophyll is the green pigment found in plants. This green pigment helps plants absorb light from the sun, this process is called photosynthesis. Chlorophyll contains many powerful nutrients, such as vitamin A, C, E, K, and beta-carotene. Chlorophyll is very high in antioxidants, and important minerals such as magnesium, iron, potassium, calcium, and essential fatty acids. Food sources include all green vegetables, chlorella and spirulina.

Collagen

Collagen is the most abundant protein found throughout the human body. It is in our connective tissue, bones, skin, muscles, cartilage, tendons, ligaments, teeth, blood vessels, and the digestive system. Collagen is what gives skin elasticity, and helps give the body form, structure, support and flexibility. Dark leafy greens, beans, carrots, garlic, citrus fruit, red berries, flaxseeds, and soy are good sources of collagen.

Cyanidin

Cyanidin is a red pigment found in red and dark colored berries and grapes. The highest concentration of cyanidin is found in the skin of these fruits. It is a natural organic compound, and has many health benefits including anti-cancer properties, improving joint health, and regulating blood sugar.

Essential Fatty Acids

The two essential fatty acids, also known as EFAs, are omega 3 (Alpha-linolenic acid) and omega 6 (linoleic acid). We cannot manufacture these fatty acids within the human body so it is essential that we acquire them through food. They have many important functions, and play a vital role in health. Balancing the ratio of omega 3 to omega 6 is also important. These EFAs work as anti-inflammatory compounds playing a role in joint health, cardiovascular health, immunity, and overall well-being. Plant sources of omega 3s include walnuts, flaxseeds, chia seeds, hemp and soy. Plant sources of omega 6 include nuts, açaí, avocado, hemp, flaxseeds, pumpkin seeds, chia seeds and sunflower seeds.

Flavonoids

Flavonoids are substances found in plants that have antioxidant capabilities. They make up the largest group of phytonutrients, over six thousand have been identified so far. Flavonoids are found in abundance in whole plant foods, especially tea, citrus fruits, and berries, along with many other fruits and vegetables.

Polyphenols

Polyphenols are micronutrients found in plant foods. They are loaded with antioxidants, and provide many different health benefits. One example of a polyphenol is resveratrol, which is well known for its anti-inflammatory ability. Polyphenols help lower blood pressure, lower cholesterol levels, and improve heart function. Sources include raw cacao, dark chocolate, cloves, star anise, elderberry, red and black grapes, dried Mexican oregano, chestnut, and ground flaxseed.

Quercetin

Quercetin, a type of polyphenol from the flavonoid group of antioxidant compounds, is a super micronutrient, and has amazing anti-inflammatory properties that may help ward off many diseases ranging from stomach inflammatory conditions to eye-related disorders. Quercetin is found in a wide range of plant foods, including peppers, berries, leafy greens, apples, citrus fruits, cranberries, buckwheat, sage, and cacao, as well as black and green teas.

Whole Foods

Whole foods are foods as close to their natural state as possible with very little removed during processing. Fruits, vegetables, beans (legumes), nuts, seeds, and whole grains are all considered whole foods.

Zeaxanthin

Zeaxanthin is one of the most powerful carotenoids found in plants, and has very important functions in the body especially when it comes to healthy vision. It performs in conjunction with lutein in protecting the retina from oxidative damage. Sources of zeaxanthin and lutein include paprika, bell peppers, saffron, green leafy vegetables, and many other colorful fruits and vegetables.

Useful Resources

Açaí Powder: Navitas

Açaí berries are rich in fatty acids, and super rich in antioxidants making them free-radical eradicators. Navitas are a high quality, organic, well trusted producer of many different superfoods.

Aloe Vera: Lily of the desert (inner fillet)

Fresh leaf is best, but this is second best. Aloe vera increases the absorption of nutrients from foods, and supports a healthy digestive system. This is a preservative-free organic aloe vera juice.

Amaranth (Organic Whole Grain): Arrowhead Mills

Amaranth is a gluten free ancient grain high in fiber and protein. Delicious as a breakfast porridge, or popped. Arrowhead Mills has been around for fifty years growing organic high-quality grains.

Beans and Lentils (Sprouted): tru Roots

Consuming sprouted beans and lentils enhances digestibility, which enables the body to absorb more nutrients. tru Roots produce nutritious and delicious organic sprouted beans and lentils.

Buckwheat: Bob's Red Mill

Organic whole grain creamy buckwheat hot cereal. This buckwheat is my favorite breakfast cereal. Gluten free, creamy and full of flavor. See my high energy breakfast recipes. Bob's Red Mill is a quality company, and producer of many different whole grains.

Cacao Butter: Terrasoul

This is my secret to holding together "Live" Raw bars. Delicious and creamy, solid at room temperature. Terrasoul organic raw cacao butter is cold-pressed and smells amazing.

Cacao Powder and Cacao Nibs: Navitas

Organic, packed with energy and antioxidants with the heavenly scent of chocolate.

Camu Camu Powder: Navitas

Camu camu is super high in vitamin C, which strengthens the immune system, and contains anti-viral properties.

Chia Seeds: There are so many great brands available, it is difficult to choose just one. So here are a few:

> Nutiva
> Healthworks
> Kiva
> Navitas

Chlorella: Microingredients

Chlorella is a complete protein superfood. Chlorella powder from Microingredients is USDA certified organic and harvested from fresh water, bright green in color with a fresh smell.

Coconut Nectar: Big Tree Farms

Coconut nectar is low on the GI (glycemic index), and high in minerals. It is also high in amino acids, and helps to balance pH. This high quality, low glycemic sweetener is delicious. Big Tree Farms coconut nectar comes from organic coconuts in Western Bali.

Goldenberries: Navitas

Goldenberries are also known as cape gooseberries. They help to decrease inflammation, are dense in antioxidants, detoxifying, and immunity boosting. Navitas are a high quality, organic, well trusted producer of many different superfoods.

Goji Berries: Navitas

Navitas are a high quality, organic, well trusted producer of many different superfoods.

Hemp: Manitoba Harvest

Manitoba Harvest are growers of a premium hemp seeds. Other products they produce include hemp oil, hemp protein powder, hemp flour, and hemp heart bites. They grow their hemp pesticide free, and organic, and retain nutrient content through minimal processing of products.

Maca Powder: Terrasoul

The highest quality maca root comes from Peru. Maca powder by Terrasoul is organic, highly digestible and bioavailable. Maca root helps the body adapt to stress, balances hormones, and increases stamina.

Matcha Green Tea: Encha

One of the highest quality organic matcha green tea powders available. Harvested from the most tender organic leaves in Japan.

Mulberries: Navitas

Mulberries aid digestion, and may help to lower cholesterol. They also increase circulation and boost bone density. Navitas are a high quality, organic, well trusted producer of many different superfoods.

Power Snacks: Navitas

These snacks are delicious and organic, and different varieties are available. I like citrus chia and coffee cacao. Great as snacks, or as toppings for chia puddings and breakfast bowls.

Pumpkin and Sunflower Seeds: Go Raw

Go Raw sells delicious and highly nutritious, organic, sprouted pumpkin and sunflowers seeds.

Pumpkin Seed Oil: Dr. Adorable

This pumpkin seed oil is organic, unrefined, and cold pressed. It is rich in vitamins A, B, D, and E, and a great source of minerals, proteins, and essential fatty acids.

Pumpkin Seed Butter: Jiva Organics

Raw, organic, and sprouted, with a delicious, creamy flavor, and easy to digest, and also higher in nutrients than un-sprouted pumpkin seed butters.

Rice: Lunberg

California rice grower, Lunberg test their products for arsenic levels, and are found to have lower levels than other brands grown in different regions of the country. They grow many different varieties of brown rice. They also grow organic wild rice, red rice, and sprouted varieties.

Sorghum: Bob's Red Mill

Sorghum has been around since Benjamin Franklin, a high fiber, gluten free grain with many health benefits.

Spirulina: Nutrex

Grown naturally in Hawaii and very high quality. An extremely nutritious superfood containing 60 percent protein.

Teff: Bob's Red Mill

Originating back thousands of years, and the traditional grain of Ethiopia. Teff is delicious as a whole grain porridge or can be popped and added to soups, stews or baked goods. It can be ground down to make flour or bought as a flour. Good source of calcium, fiber and protein.

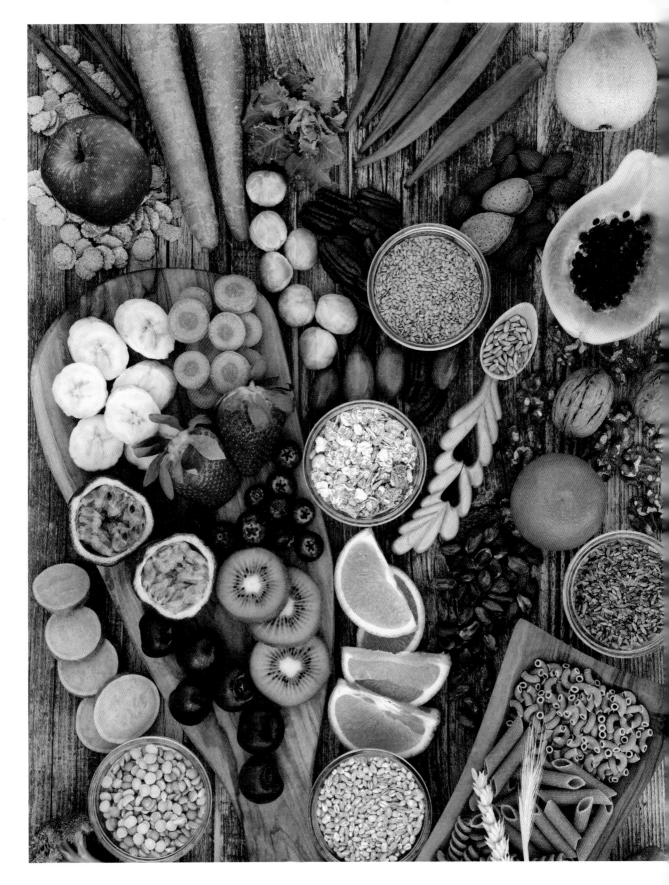

Bibliography

Andrews, Ryan. "Phytates and phytic acid: Here's what you need to know." *Precision Nutrition*, www.precisionnutrition.com/all-about-phytates-phytic-acid.

Arnarson, Atli. "Bananas 101: Nutrition Facts and Health Benefits." Healthline, 10 Oct. 2014, www.healthline.com/nutrition/foods/bananas.

"Arsenic in Rice and Rice Products Risk Assessment Report." *U.S. Food and Drug Administration*, March 2016. www.fda.gov/downloads/Food/FoodScienceResearch/RiskSafetyAssessment/UCM486543.pdf.

Barnard, Neal D., Joshua Cohen, David J.A. Jenkins, Gabrielle Turner-McGrievy, Lise Gloede, Amber Green, and Hope Ferdowsian. "A Low-Fat Vegan Diet and a Conventional Diabetes Diet in the Treatment of Type 2 Diabetes: A Randomized, Controlled, 74-Wk Clinical Trial." *The American Journal of Clinical Nutrition*, vol. 89, no. 5, 2009, pp. 1588S–1596S. *National Center for Biotechnology Information, U.S. National Library of Medicine*, www.ncbi.nlm.nih.gov/pmc/articles/PMC2677007/.

Big Tree Farms, bigtreefarms.com.

"Bisphenol A (BPA)." *National Institute of Environmental Health Sciences*, www.niehs.nih.gov/health/topics/agents/sya-bpa/index.cfm.

Bjarnadottir, Adda. "Everything you need to know about avocado," *Medical News Today*, 1 Aug. 2017, http://www.medicalnewstoday.com/articles/318620.

Bluvas, Erin. "Brie Turner-McGrievy Receives Nearly $3.3 Million NIH Grant to Reduce Heart Disease through Nutrition-Based Approach," *Arnold School of Public Health, University of South Carolina,* **17** Aug. 2017, www.sc.edu/study/colleges_schools/public_health/about/news/2017/turner-mcgrievy_grant.php#.WjRbVK2ZP-Y.

Busch, Sandi. "What Are the Benefits of Eating Red Cabbage?" *Healthy Eating,* 11 Dec. 2017, www.healthyeating.sfgate.com/benefits-eating-red-cabbage-4395.html.

Callaway, J.C. "Hempseed as a Nutritional Resource: An Overview." *Euphytica*, vol. 140, no. 1–2, Jan. 2004, pp. 65–72. *Springer Link*, link.springer.com/article/10.1007/s10681-004-4811-6.

Campbell, T. Colin. "Dietary protein, growth factors, and cancer." *The American Journal of Clinical Nutrition*, vol. 85, no. 6, 1 June 2007, p. 1667, ajcn.nutrition.org/content/85/6/1667.full.

Choudhury, K., J. Clark, and H.R. Griffiths. "An Almond-Enriched Diet Increases Plasma α-Tocopherol and Improves Vascular Function but Does Not Affect Oxidative Stress Markers or Lipid Levels." *Free Radical Research*, vol. 48, no. 5, 2014, pp. 599–606. *Taylor & Francis Online*, www.tandfonline.com/doi/abs/10.3109/10715762.2014.896458.

Colquhoun, James. "25 Powerful Reasons to Eat Bananas," *Food Matters*, 14 Aug. 2012, www.foodmatters.com/articles25-powerful-reasons-to-eat-bananas.

Cottis, Halle. *Whole Lifestyle Nutrition*, www.wholelifestylenutrition. com/phyticacid.

Dreher, Mark L., and Adrienne J. Davenport. "Hass Avocado Composition and Potential Health Effects." *Critical Reviews in Food Science and Nutrition*, vol. 53, no. 7, 2013, pp. 738– 750. *PubMed Central*, www.ncbi.nlm.nih.gov/pmc/articles/ PMC3664913/.

Esselstyn, Caldwell B., Jr., Gina Gendy, Jonathan Doyle, Mladen Golubic, and Michael F. Roizen. "A way to reverse CAD?" *The Journal of Family Practice*, vol. 63, no. 7, pp. 356–364b, July 2014, dresselstyn.com/JFP_06307_Article1.pdf.

"Exercising to relax." *Harvard Medical School*, Feb. 2011, www. health.harvard.edu/staying-healthy/exercising-to-relax.

FECYT-Spanish Foundation for Science and Technology. "Cloves Are 'Best' Natural Antioxidant, Spanish Study Finds." *ScienceDaily*, 19 Mar. 2010, www.sciencedaily.com/ releases/2010/03/100316124231.htm.

Gordon, E.C. "12 Surprising Health Benefits of Lemons and Limes." *Aviva Natural Health*, http://www.avivahealth.com/ article.asp?articleid=276.

Greger, Michael. "Harvard's Meat and Mortality Studies." *Dr. Greger's Medical Nutrition Blog*, 15 Mar. 2012, nutritionfacts. org/2012/03/15/harvards-meat-and-mortality-studies/.

Gupta, Subash C., Sridevi Patchva, and Bharat B. Aggarwal. "Therapeutic Roles of Curcumin: Lessons Learned from Clinical Trials." *The AAPS Journal*, vol. 15, no. 1, 2013, pp. 195–218. *PubMed Central*, www.ncbi.nlm.nih.gov/pmc/articles/ PMC3535097/.

Han, Emily. "7 Ways to Eat & Drink Turmeric," *The Kitchn*, 22 Sep. 2017, https://www.thekitchn. com/7-ways-to-eat-drink-turmeric-198696.

"History of Onions." *National Onion Association*, www.onions-usa. org/all-about-onions/history-of-onions.

Holick, M.F. "Vitamin D and Bone Health," *The Journal of Nutrition*, vol. 126, no. 4), 1 Apr 1996, pp. 1159S–1164S. *Europe PMC*, europepmc.org/abstract/MED/8642450/reload=0;jsessionid=C WDKSTTukTs192guwz6e.8.

"How Spices Shaped History." *The Spice Trader*, www. thespicetrader.co.nz/history-of-spice/.

Isa, Joan. "Hiatal Hernia, GERD, Indigestion." *Dr. McDougall's Health and Medical Center.* www.drmcdougall.com/health/education/ health-science/stars/stars-written/joan-isa/.

Isaacs, Tony. "Amazing health benefits of parsley, sage, rosemary and thyme." Align Life, https://alignlife.com/articles/antiaging/ amazing-health-benefits-of-parsley-sage-rosemary-and-tyme.

Jenkins, David J.A., Cyril W.C. Kendall, Augustine Marchie, Tina L. Parker, Philip W. Connelly, Wei Qian, James S. Haight, Dorothea Faulkner, Edward Vidgen, Karen G. Lapsley, and Gene A. Spiller. "Dose Response of Almonds on Coronary Heart Disease Risk Factors: Blood Lipids, Oxidized Low-Density Lipoproteins, Lipoprotein(a), Homocysteine, and Pulmonary Nitric Oxide." *Circulation*, vol. 106, 2002, pp. 1327–1332, circ.ahajournals.org/content/106/11/1327.short.

Karkos, P.D., S. C. Leong, C. D. Karkos, N. Sivaji, and D.A. Assimakopoulos. "*Spirulina* in Clinical Practice: Evidence-Based Human Applications." *Evidence-Based Complementary and Alternative Medicine*, 2011. *PubMed Central*, 28 Mar. 2018, www.ncbi.nlm.nih.gov/pmc/articles/PMC3136577/.

Leech, Joe. "10 Proven Health Benefits of Blueberries." *Healthline*, 4 June 2017, www.healthline.com/ nutrition/10-proven-benefits-of-blueberries.

——. "11 Proven Health Benefits of Garlic." *Healthline*, 19 Jan. 2017, www.healthline.com/nutrition/11-proven-benefits-of-garlic.

——. "11 Proven Health Benefits of Ginger." *Healthline*, 4 June 2017, www.healthline.com/nutrition/11-proven-benefits-of-ginger.

Lisker, R. and L. Aguilar. "Double Blind Study of Milk Lactose Intolerance." *Gastroenterology*, vol. 74, no. 6, June 1978, pp. 1283–1285. *PubMed Central*, www.ncbi.nlm.nih.gov/pubmed/348553.

Live Science, www.livescience.com.

Masterjohn, Chris. "The Truth about the China Study." *cholesterol-and-health.com*, http://www.cholesterol-and-health.com/China-Study.html.

"The McDougall Program Cohort: The Largest Study of the Benefits from a Medical Dietary Intervention." *Dr. McDougall's Health and Medical Center*, 2014, www.drmcdougall.com/2014/10/31/the-mcdougall-program-cohort-the-largest-study-of-the-benefits-from-a-medical-dietary-intervention/.

Merchant, R.E., and C.A. Andre. "A Review of Recent Clinical Trials of the Nutritional Supplement Chlorella pyrenoidosa in the Treatment of Fibromyalgia, Hypertension, and Ulcerative Colitis." *Alternative Therapies in Health and Medicine*, vol. 7, no. 3, May–June 2001, pp. 79–91. *PubMed Central*, www.ncbi.nlm.nih.gov/pubmed/11347287.

Mercola, Joseph. "9 Health Benefits of Pumpkin Seeds," *Mercola*, 30 Sept. 2013, articles.mercola.com/sites/articles/archive/2013/09/30/pumpkin-seed-benefits.aspx.

Muthaiyah, Balu, Musthafa M. Essa, Moon Lee, Ved Chauhan, Kulbir Kaur, and Abha Chauhan. "Dietary Supplementation of Walnuts Improves Memory Deficits and Learning Skills in Transgenic Mouse Model of Alzheimer's Disease," *Journal of Alzheimer's Disease*, vol. 42, no. 4, 2014, pp. 1397–1405. *IOS Press*, content.iospress.com/articles/journal-of-alzheimers-disease/jad140675.

"Nutmeg." *Encyclopædia Britannica*, 6 Dec. 2017, www.britannica.com/topic/nutmeg.

Olney, J.W. "Excitotoxins in foods." *Neurotoxicology*, vol. 15, no. 3, Fall 1994, pp. 535–544. *Europe PMC*, europepmc.org/abstract/med/7854587.

Ornish, Dean, Larry W. Scherwitz, James H. Billings, K. Lance Gould, Terri A. Merritt, Stephen Sparler, William T. Armstrong, Thomas A. Ports, Richard L. Kirkeeide, Charissa Hogeboom, Richard J. "Intensive Lifestyle Changes for Reversal of Coronary Heart Disease." *Journal of the American Medical Association*, vol. 280, no. 23, 16 Dec. 1998, pp. 2001–2007. *Ornish Lifestyle Medicine*, www.ornish.com/wp-content/uploads/Intensive-lifestyle-changes-for-reversal-of-coronary-heart-disease1.pdf.

"Paleo Diet Is Dangerous, Increases Weight Gain, Diabetes Expert Warns." *ScienceDaily*, 18 Feb. 2016, www.sciencedaily.com/releases/2016/02/160218114753.htm.

Pannunzio, Lu Ann. "5 of the Best Matcha Green Tea Brands Out There." The Cup of Life, https://theteacupoflife.com/2015/10/5-of-best-matcha-green-tea-brands-out.html.

Paris, Phillip. "Goji Berries: Origins—Consumption—Nutrition Facts—Health Benefits." *NutritiousFruit.com*, http://www.nutritiousfruit.com/goji-berries.html.

Park, Sung-Woo, Joo-Young Kim, You-Sun Kim, Sang Jin Lee, Sang Don Lee, and Moon Kee Chung. "A Milk Protein, Casein, as a Proliferation Promoting Factor in Prostate Cancer Cells." *The World Journal of Men's Health*, vol. 32, no. 2, 2014, pp. 76–82. PubMed Central, www.ncbi.nlm.nih.gov/pmc/articles/PMC4166373/.

"Parsley." *Our Herb Garden*, www.ourherbgarden.com/herb-history/parsley.html.

Rao, Pasupuleti Visweswara and Siew Hua Gan. "Cinnamon: A Multifaceted Medicinal Plant." *Evidence-based Complementary and Alternative Medicine*, 10 Apr. 2014. *PubMed Central*, www.ncbi.nlm.nih.gov/pmc/articles/PMC4003790/.

Rayment, W.J. "The Health Effects of Nutmeg." *InDepthInfo.com*, www.indepthinfo.com/nutmeg/health-effects.shtml.

Reschke, Glenn. "Learn Here about the Historical Uses of Cayenne Pepper," *Your Cayenne Pepper Guide*, www.cayennepepper.info/historical-uses-of-cayenne-pepper.html.

Rink, Lothar. "Zinc and the Immune System." *Proceedings of the Nutrition Society*, vol. 59, no. 4, 2000, pp. 541–552, doi.org/10.1017/S0029665100000781.

Robertson, Ruairi. "Why the Gut Microbiome Is Crucial for Your Health." *Healthline*, 27 June 2017, www.healthline.com/nutrition/gut-microbiome-and-health.

Roseboro, Ken. "Scientist's Ground-Breaking Research Uncovers New Risks of GMOs, Glyphosate." *The Organic & Non-GMO Report*, 26 Jan. 2017, non-gmoreport.com/articles/scientists-ground-breaking-research-uncovers-new-risks-gmos-glyphosate/.

Rudrappa, Umesh. "Cloves nutrition facts." *Nutrition and You*, www.nutrition-and-you.com/cloves.html.

Shaw, Jonathan. "A Diabetes Link to Meat," *Harvard Magazine*, Jan.–Feb. 2012, www.harvardmagazine.com/2012/01/a-diabetes-link-to-meat.

Surjushe, Amar, Resham Vasani, and D.G. Saple. "Aloe Vera: A Short Review." *Indian Journal of Dermatology*, vol. 53, no. 4, 2008, pp. 163–166. *PubMed Central*, www.ncbi.nlm.nih.gov/pmc/articles/PMC2763764/.

Urbano, G., M. López-Jurado, P. Aranda, C. Vidal-Valverde, E. Tenorio, and J. Porres. "The Role of Phytic Acid in Legumes:

Antinutrient or Beneficial Function?" *Journal of Physiology and Biochemistry*, vol. 56, 2000, pp. 283–294. *PubMed* Central, www.ncbi.nlm.nih.gov/pubmed/11198165.

Ware, Megan. "Everything You Need to Know about Blueberries." *Medical News Today*, 5 Sept. 2017, www.medicalnewstoday.com/articles/287710.php.

——. "Is Matcha Good for You, and How Can You Use It?" *Medical News Today*, 19 Oct. 2017, www.medicalnewstoday.com/articles/305289.php.

——. "What's to know about sweet potatoes?" *Medical News Today*, 1 Sept. 2017, www.medicalnewstoday.com/articles/281438.php.

"Watercress: The Powerhouse Vegetable That Fights Chronic Diseases." *Axe Wellness*, http://draxe.com/watercress/.

"What's so healthy about basil?" *Spezzatino Magazine*, vol. 7. *Healthy Food Bank Foundation*, www.precisionnutrition.com/healthy-basil.

Wien, M.A., J.M. Sabaté, D.N. Iklé, S.E. Cole, and F.R. Kandeel. "Almonds vs. Complex Carbohydrates in a Weight Reduction Program," *International Journal of Obesity*, vol. 27, 2003, pp. 1365–1372. *Nature.com*, www.nature.com/ijo/journal/v27/n11/abs/0802411a.html.

"Yoga for Anxiety and Depression." *Harvard Medical School*, 18 Sept. 2017, www.health.harvard.edu/mind-and-mood/yoga-for-anxiety-and-depression.

"You Can Learn a Lot from a Label." *Self*, nutritiondata.self.com.

Zavala, Yamily J., and John M. Duxbury. "Arsenic in Rice: I. Estimating Normal Levels of Total Arsenic in Rice Grain." *Environmental Science & Technology*, vol. 42, no. 10, 15 May 2008, pp. 3856–3860. *American Chemical Society*, pubs.acs.org/doi/abs/10.1021/es702747y.

Recipe Index

291

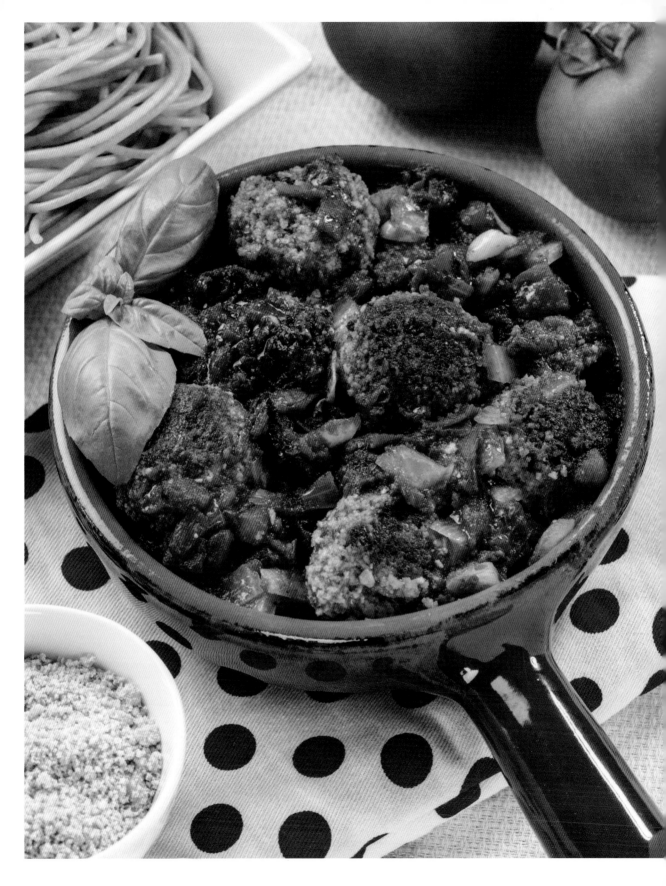

Subject Index

Page numbers in *italics* denote charts or figures.